LACTIVISM

LACTIVISM

HOW **FEMINISTS** AND **FUNDAMENTALISTS,**
HIPPIES AND **YUPPIES,** AND **PHYSICIANS**
AND **POLITICIANS** MADE **BREASTFEEDING**
BIG BUSINESS AND **BAD POLICY**

COURTNEY JUNG

BASIC BOOKS
A Member of the Perseus Books Group
New York

Published by Basic Books,
A Member of the Perseus Books Group

Books published by Basic Books are available at special discounts
for bulk purchases in the United States by corporations, institutions,
and other organizations. For more information, please contact the
Special Markets Department at the Perseus Books Group,
2300 Chestnut Street, Suite 200, Philadelphia, PA 19103,
or call (800) 810-4145, ext. 5000,
or e-mail special.markets@perseusbooks.com.

Designed by Cynthia Young

Library of Congress Cataloging-in-Publication Data
Jung, Courtney, 1965–
Lactivism : how feminists and fundamentalists, hippies and yuppies, and
physicians and politicians made breastfeeding big business and bad policy /
Courtney Jung.—First Edition.
pages cm
Includes bibliographical references and index.
ISBN 978-0-465-03969-2 (hardback)—ISBN 978-0-465-06165-5 (e-book)
1. Women's studies—United States. 2. Breastfeeding—Social aspects—
United States. 3. Infants—Nutrition—United States. I. Title.
HQ1181.U5J86 2015
305.40973—dc23
2015011122

10 9 8 7 6 5 4 3 2 1

For Serena and Peter, my inspiration

Contents

Introduction

Yummy Mummy is a small store in the middle of a quietly commercial block of Manhattan's Lexington Avenue. Flanked by a dog accessory store and a beauty salon, it is surrounded by expensive boutiques specializing in children. A quick glance reveals a children's optician, a children's photographer, a handful of children's clothing stores, and a nanny agency. Tastefully decorated and brimming with designer apparel and accessories for nursing mothers, Yummy Mummy fits right in. Its plum brown awning greets customers and passers-by with a friendly, if pointed, message: *happy breastfeeding*.

Located on the Upper East Side, just one block away from the mansions and penthouses of Park Avenue, Yummy Mummy is a self-styled "breastfeeding emporium." A steady stream of new mothers pushing state-of-the-art strollers flock here to buy everything from bottles and bras to "hip, stylish" nursing clothes and breastfeeding supplements like Lactation Cookies. As it happens, Lactation Cookies look just like ordinary chocolate-chip cookies, but they include ingredients such as oats, brewers' yeast, and flax seed to boost breast-milk production. (Yummy Mummy also sells fenugreek for the same purpose, which at ten dollars a package, costs half the price.)

Still, Yummy Mummy's main business is breast pumps, which it sells at the small Lexington Avenue store and through its bustling website. Although breast pump sales have been brisk ever since Amanda Cole opened her store in 2009, they soared dramatically in 2013. That year, President Obama made a bold intervention in the world of breastfeeding advocacy by reforming the Affordable Care Act (ACA) to require health insurance companies to cover the cost of breast pumps for new mothers. At first, Cole worried that making breast pumps free to anyone with health insurance would be bad for business. Even before the ACA reform went into effect, the United States accounted for 40 percent of the global market in breast pumps, with 2.3 million breast pumps sold in 2010 alone. After the reform, analysts predicted the breast pump market would expand by 50 percent, and Cole didn't want to miss out on that burgeoning growth.

She moved quickly to make the new legislation work to her advantage. Insurance companies will only reimburse customers who purchase equipment through an accredited durable medical equipment (DME) supplier. These specialized stores normally sell institutional items like hospital beds and oxygen tanks; their no-nonsense aesthetic is light years away from the boutique-y world of Yummy Mummy. But, by deftly navigating the bureaucracy necessary to have Yummy Mummy accredited as a DME, Cole positioned her store to profit from the new plan almost immediately. Only months after the breast pump benefit went into effect, consumer demand had soared to the point that she hired an additional seventeen workers and rented space for a call center to handle the national orders coming through the store's website.

Yummy Mummy now has established relationships with twenty-five different insurance plans and ships hundreds of pumps per week. Industry analysts expect this market to grow even more, as news of the benefit spreads. By the end of the decade, the American breast-pump market should reach almost one billion dollars—and the market for the other breastfeeding equipment Yummy Mummy sells, including clothes, bras, creams, and pillows, will be roughly double that.

With a little help from President Obama's Affordable Care Act, breastfeeding has become very big business indeed.

LIKE SO MANY LIFESTYLE COMPANIES TODAY, from Whole Foods to the Arbor Collective skateboard company, Yummy Mummy is a compelling mixture of conscience and commerce, an enterprise dedicated to doing well by doing good. As a new mother in Manhattan, Cole was committed to breastfeeding but frustrated by the absence of good breastfeeding products and informed advice. Ultimately, that frustration exposed a market opportunity. Her neighborhood needed a place that would cater to, and support, nursing women. In 2009, Cole opened a store she envisioned as a one-stop shop for premium breastfeeding products and a community hub where expectant or new parents could consult well-informed sales associates—including Cole herself, who is now a certified lactation counselor. The store also offers a range of courses. There are standard offerings such as "Childbirth Preparation" and "Baby Safety & CPR" and less standard offerings such as "Eat, Drink, Doula." Billed as a form of "speed dating," "Eat, Drink, Doula" streamlines parents' search for a labor coach by introducing them to five to ten prospective doulas in a single session.

The consumer culture that has grown up around breastfeeding says a great deal about its core demographic, its lifestyle priorities, and the resources it has to dedicate to breastfeeding. As its cheeky name suggests, Yummy Mummy's mission is not confined to the worthy causes of infant and maternal health and environmental and economic well-being mentioned on its website. In contemporary slang, a yummy mummy is a sexy, glamorous mother—well dressed and, usually, well heeled too. Tabloids use the term to praise celebrity moms like Miranda Kerr and Angelina Jolie for refusing to let motherhood cramp their fabulous lifestyles—and wardrobes. Yummy Mummy too signals that breastfeeding is no longer just for the crunchy earth-mother crowd. Along with breast pumps and vitamins, the store offers all the trendy fashion items and accessories a mother needs to "nurse in style." Breastfeeding is the new black.

At this moment in the long history of infant feeding, when maternity and breastfeeding boutiques with whimsical names— like The Pumping Station in Santa Monica or Manhattan's Upper Breast Side—have multiplied in desirable zip codes around the country, it's worth remembering that the very idea of "nursing in style" marks a dramatic cultural shift. Not very long ago, the idea of breastfeeding stylishly would have seemed patently absurd. Back in the 1970s, many of the women who revived the practice of breastfeeding in the US were making a political statement, not a fashion statement. They were taking a stand for women's right to choose how to feed their babies, and against big businesses like Nestlé that were peddling formula in poor countries at the expense of babies' lives. But the mainstreaming of breastfeeding has generated not only countless bad puns—a nursing pillow called My Breast Friend, a postpartum girdle called the Mother Tucker—it has also stimulated a booming market in luxury breastfeeding paraphernalia that the earlier generation of feminists, hippies, and countercultural mavericks could never have imagined.

One of the most popular electric pumps in the US, manufactured by the Swiss company Medela, is called the Pump in Style. Anyone even remotely familiar with the mechanics of breast pumping will find the idea of pumping in style amusing, at best. Naked from the waist up, with suction cups attached to each swollen nipple as the pump yanks loudly and rhythmically to coax milk into plastic cylinders, not even Heidi Klum could look stylish. But the name is telling nonetheless. It bespeaks an ideal of motherhood that is alluring to many women—and profitable to the many manufacturers and stores that promise ways of achieving it.

The trappings of contemporary breastfeeding culture—including breast pumps, designer apparel from companies with names like Boob and Glamourmom, and Lactation Cookies—reflect the tangled web of social, political, and commercial interests that sustain it. This new culture—at once wholesome and hip—is partly the result of a hard-won social pride. Many of those who revived breastfeeding in the twentieth century—feminists, hippies, and members of La Leche League included—encountered considerable resistance. And some still do. Sometimes these tensions are generational and subtle. New mothers who breastfeed often report that their own mothers, who didn't, are critical and defensive. *After all, you turned out all right, didn't you?*

Other times the resistance is not subtle at all. To this day, women are harassed for breastfeeding in public at places as diverse as Friendly's Restaurant, Target, and Anthropologie clothing store. When seen in this light, the new generation of breastfeeding advocates' emphasis on style can be seen as an important effort to show that breastfeeding and motherhood are compatible with having a life—a life that doesn't rule out fitness, fashion, and fun. This is an undeniably good cause.

The many initiatives designed to protect a woman's right to breastfeed in public represent a similarly worthy expression of female pride. In fact, this particular right has recently become, quite literally, a cause célèbre. Famous mothers like Kourtney Kardashian, Gwen Stefani, and Maggie Gyllenhaal have all made a point of being photographed nursing in public. As with gay rights and other identity-based political movements, their strategy is to embrace visibility as a way of refusing stigma and shame. In 2015, even Pope Francis weighed in, encouraging mothers to nurse their babies during a baptismal ceremony in the Sistine Chapel.

More formally organized initiatives exist now too. Started several years ago in New Zealand, the Big Latch On has become a global event in which women come together to breastfeed in public, en masse, on a given day in the beginning of August, during World Breastfeeding Week. The advocacy organization Best for Babes runs a national hotline for mothers who are harassed for nursing in public. The phone number is 855-NIP-FREE. And then there's one of the most colorful citizen initiatives, The Milk Truck, a big pink van with a three-foot-high fiberglass breast and flashing nipple on its roof that rescues women in Pittsburgh who are harassed for breastfeeding in public.

Initiatives like the Big Latch On and The Milk Truck strike me as positive examples of breastfeeding advocacy. Their goal is to protect women's ability to choose how and where to feed their children. But as I've discovered again and again while writing this book, breastfeeding advocacy too often crosses the line into lactivism, including compulsory breastfeeding, breastfeeding as a moral crusade, and breastfeeding as a means of distinguishing good from bad parents. When it does, it *limits* rather than *protects* women's choices. Some lactivists have in fact described "choice" as the language of the enemy. Their campaigns are specifically designed to undermine the idea that women can take into account their own individual circumstances—jobs, child-care options, and so on—when choosing how to feed their babies. At their most extreme, lactivists view breastfeeding as an end in itself—an activity to be defended at all costs, even when it threatens the health and well-being of babies and mothers.

Not long ago, the supermodel Gisele Bündchen displayed an unexpected flair for policy reform when she called for a "worldwide law" requiring women to breastfeed for six months. In Saudi Arabia, women *are* legally obligated to breastfeed—for two years. Here in the US, politicians and policy makers have stopped short of legislating breastfeeding, but they have decided that breastfeeding should be viewed as a matter of public policy rather than a personal choice. Since 2010, the Centers for Disease Control and Prevention (CDC), the American Academy of Pediatrics (AAP), and the US Surgeon General have all officially identified breastfeeding as "a public health issue." This declaration places formula feeding on a par with smoking and unsafe sex as a form of risky behavior that threatens not only individual health but American society at large. As Dr. Richard Schanler, the chair of the AAP Section on Breastfeeding, explained in an interview, "This is a health issue for the better health of our infants, so why are we just leaving it up to the whim of the family to do whatever they feel like?"

In fact, so many people agree with Schanler and Bündchen these days that breastfeeding has become what political scientists like me identify as a consensus issue—an issue
that unites people who otherwise disagree about pretty much
everything else. Feminists and fundamentalists, yuppies and
hippies, conservatives and liberals, the medical establishment
and its alternative-medicine critics: for all their differences,
they are all aligned on this particular issue. The problem is
that these unlikely bedfellows not only believe in breastfeeding and practice it themselves; they often believe that every-
body else should too. Breastfeeding is no longer just a way to
feed a baby; it is a moral marker that distinguishes *us* from
them—good parents from bad.

For many well-educated middle- and upper-middle-class
parents, breastfeeding is an early foray into competitive parenting. They breastfeed because it promises to produce children
who are healthier, more secure, and smarter. In these circles,
breastfeeding is also an indicator of financial or professional
success—only mothers who have the luxury of time or job flex-
ibility can breastfeed long enough to claim the full health benefits. In the United States today, breastfeeding is undeniably a
marker of class status, although not for everyone. For the Christian right, the value of breastfeeding is different. Fundamentalist Christians cite scripture to show that breastfeeding is part of
God's plan. It also offers proof of intelligent design—the theory
that the universe was created by God's design rather than the
big bang and evolution—and it signals womanly submission
to God's will. Ironically, breastfeeding means just the oppo-
site to feminists, for whom it is often a form of empowerment
that offers evidence of the life-sustaining force of female bodies. For the hippie and hipster left, breastfeeding is also a moral

imperative, though here too, for different reasons. Hipsters breastfeed because they are environmentalists, because they support the local food movement, and because they are critical of the huge multinationals that make formula. Breastfeeding is part of a package of lifestyle choices that will often include yoga, farmers' markets, fair-trade coffee, cloth diapers, and home-made baby food. If you find yourself feeding your baby formula at the Food Co-op in Park Slope, you may as well be wearing a coat made of baby sealskins.

The moral righteousness surrounding breastfeeding has been bolstered by claims that formula feeding not only imposes costs on babies but on society as a whole. In 2010, the medical journal *Pediatrics* published an article claiming that the failure to breastfeed was costing the United States $13 billion per year in health-care costs, infant deaths, and the lost lifetime earnings of those dead babies. And that number would be higher still, the article continued, if it factored in the savings that would result from the lifelong health benefits of breastfeeding. According to the article, these benefits include "a reduction in parental absenteeism from work or adult deaths from diseases acquired in childhood."

As I elaborate in this book, such claims have been used to support interventions like Latch On NYC, a high-profile breast-feeding campaign that required New York City hospitals to keep formula under lock and key, like a prescription, and obligated new mothers who wanted to use formula to provide a medical reason for needing it. Health officials were explicit about the fact that the campaign was designed to make it harder for nurses and mothers to access formula. Many parents objected that the policy was both punitive and invasive. One mother used her own experience as an example. She could not safely

breastfeed because she was taking medication for a mental illness she did not want to discuss in her busy, shared hospital
room. Finally, after persistent questioning, she told the nurse
that, under HIPAA patient privacy provisions, she was not required to disclose that information.

But the claim that formula feeding imposes societal costs
has justified even more invasive measures in the case of poor
women. Mothers who are entitled to receive benefits from the
Special Supplemental Nutrition Program for Women, Infants,
and Children (WIC) come under sustained pressure to breastfeed. In concrete terms, WIC's decision to adopt breastfeeding
as its highest priority has meant that mothers who breastfeed
are eligible to receive WIC food benefits for twice as long as
women who use formula, and that they also receive a wider array of better food choices. Once they start eating, the babies of
breastfeeding mothers also receive more, and better, food.

Still, WIC's punitive policy was not the most extreme example of lactivism I discovered in the course of writing this
book. The most shocking example is the widespread refusal
to admit that HIV can be transmitted through breastfeeding.
Evidence that breastfeeding can transmit HIV was first published in 1985, and it has been confirmed in literally millions
of cases since then. But global public health officials ignored
that evidence for thirteen years because they feared it would
derail their breastfeeding advocacy programs. When organizations like the World Health Organization and UNICEF finally changed their policies to acknowledge that risk, some
committed lactivists, including one of the founding mothers
of La Leche League, changed tactics by joining AIDS denialists
in their claim that there is no evidence that HIV is transmitted through breastfeeding. In Chapter 7, I describe my shock

at learning that La Leche League continues to take a similarly contrarian position with respect to HIV and breastfeeding. This extreme form of lactivism, espoused by the largest and most influential breastfeeding advocacy organization in the world, is quite literally deadly.

Surprisingly, the question of choice, which is central to so many women's issues, most notably abortion, is almost totally absent from discussions about infant-feeding practices. What about women's right to choose *not* to breastfeed? Long gone are the days when breastfeeding was an act of countercultural defiance, challenging the mainstream; a right that women needed to protect at all costs. In this new era, many breastfeeding advocates—and lactivists in particular—are undermining women's right to choose in very significant ways.

The sense of moral urgency that surrounds breastfeeding advocacy creates the impression that breastfeeding has not yet caught on, that women still just don't get why it is important, and that we, as a society, are failing at this important enterprise. Yet the fact is that breastfeeding rates in the US meet or exceed the goals set out by the CDC: 79 percent of women initiate breastfeeding; 49 percent are still breastfeeding at six months.

But it is also true that breastfeeding rates are higher among white, married, well-educated, and affluent women who do not work than they are among poor women, especially African Africans, who do. As I explain in Chapter 4, the breastfeeding imperative exacerbates divisions between these two groups by elevating the infant-feeding practices of one privileged demographic—white, married, well-educated, middle-class women who stay home with their children or have flexible jobs—to the status of a national standard. Measured by this standard, the affluent white women who follow the official recommendation to breastfeed exclusively for six months are beyond reproach, both good parents and good citizens. Measured by this same standard however, the largely poor African American women who do *not* breastfeed appear to be failing in some important respect. Their decisions not to breastfeed have attracted special scrutiny, often expressed as concern.

The role of breastfeeding in aggravating long-standing American divisions of race and class came to light unexpectedly in the aftermath of Hurricane Sandy, which hit some of New York City's poorest neighborhoods particularly hard. In the kind of outpouring of goodwill that often accompanies disasters, many people volunteered to help out in those stricken neighborhoods, driving in food, cleaning up streets and devastated homes, and volunteering in temporary shelters. Bethany Yarrow, the daughter of Peter Yarrow of Peter, Paul, and Mary fame and a graduate of Yale University, was volunteering along with other mothers from the private school her children attend, and she was later interviewed about her experience by the *New York Times*.

Witness to so much devastation, in which thousands of people had lost their homes and everything they owned, Yarrow seemed especially horrified to find herself handing out cans of baby formula. According to the *New York Times*, "She was shocked by the many poor mothers in the Arverne section of the Rockaways who did not breast feed." Seventy-five percent of the population of Arverne is African American. Almost 80 percent have no education beyond high school. Meanwhile, Yarrow and her friends were working on getting a lactation consultant out to the Rockaways as soon as possible, "So that it's not just 'Here are some diapers and then go back to your misery.'" No doubt Yarrow and her friends were well intentioned, but from their position of relative privilege, breastfeeding loomed so large that it may have eclipsed any reasonable evaluation of what the women and infants of Arverne might actually need in the aftermath of a devastating storm.

Other recent US government initiatives to promote breast-feeding reinforce the message that breastfeeding is an important public policy matter. Besides the free breast pumps women are now entitled to through insurance, since 2010 the Fair Labor Standards Act has required employers "to provide reasonable break time for an employee to express breast milk for her nursing child for one year after the child's birth each time such employee has need to express milk."

As I explain in Chapter 5, these policy reforms have been celebrated as woman and breastfeeding friendly. Almost nobody talks about the fact that they are not designed to promote *breastfeeding* at all, at least as that term has traditionally been understood. They are designed to promote *pumping*. These much-touted reforms are in fact business-friendly work-arounds designed to reconcile the official recommendation that women breastfeed exclusively for six months with the fact that the US is the one country in the developed world with no paid, federally mandated maternity leave. (Women in France get sixteen weeks of leave at full pay. Women in Norway get forty-two.) Most American working mothers cobble together a combination of sick and vacation days to take six weeks of leave after the birth of a baby. But fully 30 percent of them take no maternity leave at all. And even though women now have a legal "right" to break times that will allow them to pump breast milk at work, those pumping breaks are unpaid. Such business-friendly breastfeeding initiatives sustain a lean business model by making women work harder, under greater pressure, for less money.

Policies that encourage women to pump breast milk not only step up the pressure on women, they are stealthily blurring our understanding of what breastfeeding *is*. Over the last decade in particular, the market for pumps has grown so much that manufacturers now estimate that about 85 percent of American women who breastfeed will pump. For most American mothers today, breastfeeding is accomplished, at least in part, by pumping, so that somebody else can feed their baby breast milk from a bottle while they are at work. That new norm has a wide range of unacknowledged but important implications.

First and foremost, it has shifted our understanding not only of what breastfeeding is but also how it benefits children. For decades, it was assumed that one of the primary benefits of breastfeeding was the mother-child bonding it made possible. Even when scientists began to enumerate its medical benefits, the emotional benefits of breastfeeding were also routinely emphasized. Many leading physicians and researchers continue to believe that this intimate physical contact is key. And yet, as I show in Chapter 6, the most prominent "breastfeeding" initiatives in place today focus on the chemical properties of human milk. Mother and infant bonding seems to play an increasingly minor role. In fact, the pervasive use of pumps has transformed human milk into a highly sought-after and valuable commodity, independent of its source. Thousands of people buy and sell breast milk online every day. Mostly they use it to feed their babies.

But demand for breast milk now extends beyond the pedestrian purpose of infant feeding. Human milk has become a new kind of superfood. A company called Prolacta Bioscience uses human milk to make nutritional supplements. Athletes have reportedly started drinking breast milk to boost their performance. Sometimes people with cancer give breast milk a try. Breast milk has also entered the artisanal food market. New York chef Daniel Angerer made a cheese he called Mommy's Milk from his wife's breast milk. It looked like goat's cheese and he said it tasted surprisingly sweet. It was served crusted in maple-caramelized pumpkin seeds.

At its root, the contemporary craze for human milk relies on a simple, compelling premise: that breast milk confers significant individual health advantages that collectively benefit society as a whole. For years, researchers, physicians, and breastfeeding advocates have credited breastfeeding with a dazzling array of health advantages—reducing risks for ear infections, gastrointestinal infections, lower respiratory tract infections, necrotizing enterocolitis, high blood pressure, obesity, cardiovascular disease, diabetes, asthma, allergies, cancer, celiac disease, Crohn's disease, eczema, infant mortality, and sudden infant death syndrome (SIDS), and increasing intelligence.

That simple premise informed the AAP's decision to declare breastfeeding a public health issue. It informed the Latch On NYC campaign. It is the reason for WIC's two-tiered food schedule. And it also sustains a multibillion-dollar industry devoted to breastfeeding products and accessories: an industry that has received significant support from government initiatives.

But what if that simple, compelling premise is wrong?

This book began with the sinking realization that much of the research that has justified heavy-handed public policies to promote breastfeeding is in fact outdated and characterized as "weak" by scientific standards. Different studies have reached different conclusions, yielding results that are "mixed" or "inconclusive." The most recent research, published in mainstream and highly respected journals like the *Journal of the American Medical Association, Pediatrics,* and the *British Medical Journal,* is better designed and generally considered more reliable. Many of those studies have found that breastfeeding probably has no impact on many of the health outcomes it has been associated with, or that its impact is positive but "modest." In Chapter 3, I provide a much fuller account of what researchers mean exactly by "modest." For now, let me just warn anyone who, like me, has put in countless hours nursing: it's not very encouraging.

These new research findings also cast the moral urgency surrounding breastfeeding advocacy in a new light. That passion was at least understandable when medical research depicted breastfeeding and breast milk as a magic bullet that reduced the risk of everything from cancer to obesity. But now that many of these claims are known to be unfounded, that moral passion is bewildering—and troubling.

THE TRUTH IS I BARELY THOUGHT ABOUT breastfeeding until I was thirty-nine years old and pregnant with my first child. I was surprised, delighted—and overwhelmed. I had spent almost twenty years working hard in jobs I loved, with almost complete freedom. I worked when I wanted to, which for me was pretty much all the time; I traveled; I hung out with my friends. As a graduate student and then an assistant professor, I didn't have much in the way of luxury goods, but I was luxuriously independent.

Of course, none of this prepared me for life as a pregnant woman or new mother at all. Never once had I considered what my parenting philosophy would be, or whether I would have one. Not only did I not know what the options were, I had no idea that the routines and practices of the parents I knew were part of something as coherent as a philosophy. Ferber-izing? Cosleeping? I hadn't heard of either of them. Nor did I have any idea that my friend, who breastfed each of her kids for over two years and slept in the same bed with all three of them, was practicing attachment parenting. I assumed she was practicing *birth control*.

I had a lot to learn.

Luckily for me, I was suddenly surrounded by women— friend, colleagues, acquaintances—with information and opinions they were eager to share. As I got more visibly pregnant, even women I didn't know were keen to share. I began to think of my expanding belly as a portal to a parallel universe. And in that parallel universe, breastfeeding was not only a way to feed a baby, as I had assumed before I got pregnant. It was a calling, a mission, an expression of one's deepest commitments, and a measure of one's moral worth. It wasn't just something a woman might do; it was something she believed in and even preached.

I was introduced to this sense of calling one evening at a cocktail party when I was about five months pregnant. As I looked around the room at the many people I knew, all happily sipping their pink cosmopolitans, I felt a little lightheaded and unsteady, and it didn't help that I was stone cold sober. I really wanted to go home, but it was seven o'clock. I'd just arrived.

When I saw a woman heading toward me, I welcomed the distraction. I knew her only slightly, from parties just like this one. She congratulated me on being pregnant, and I had the impression she was taking me under her wing in a maternal sort of way. But it soon became clear that she was on a serious mission to make sure that I would breastfeed my baby. She told me how important breastfeeding was for mother-child bonding and about its many medical benefits. She told me, too, about how disappointing it was that so many African American women were still not breastfeeding. I responded in what I imagined to be a reassuring manner. *"Yes, well, I'll probably breastfeed."* But obviously I wasn't reassuring enough because she kept on talking.

I picture that evening now as an awkward tango, with me repeatedly stepping backward, in retreat, while she kept advancing, all the while gesticulating dramatically with her cosmopolitan. This unlikely pas de deux stopped only when we quite literally hit a wall. We were in a corner of the yellow wallpapered kitchen with no other guests in sight. I remember thinking, "What is she *doing*?" I couldn't fathom why she cared so passionately about how I fed my baby.

But her lecture got me thinking.

Why does breastfeeding carry so much moral weight, and how much of that weight is just baggage? Are we, as mothers and as a society, investing too much in breastfeeding? And, if so, why? Even before my baby was born, encounters like the one I had at that cocktail party exposed a righteousness that made me uneasy.

Still, I breastfed my daughter. Why? Because even though I didn't want to embrace breastfeeding as an identity, or cling to it as a religion, I did want to do everything in my power to keep my baby healthy and safe. At that point I believed, as I had been told, that the medical benefits associated with breastfeeding were significant. In the end, that's all that mattered. I would breastfeed my daughter—I just wouldn't let my decision become a moral crusade. I thought of breastfeeding as a personal choice. I was a woman who happened to breastfeed and who believed in its benefits. But I was not a lactivist. I didn't think that everyone else in the world should necessarily breastfeed their babies too.

As it turned out, breastfeeding was easy for me. My tiny daughter latched like a pro so it was also the path of least resistance—even more so, when she began eating solids but still flatly refused a bottle. For months I ran home from work to feed my baby in the middle of the day, unbuttoning and rebuttoning my shirt so often I was never sure I was completely dressed. Would I say this was a good plan? *No.* Was it a plan at all? *No,* again. But unlike me, my daughter had very strong feelings about breastfeeding and a much stronger will. By the time she was two years old, and I had slowed down to a few feedings in the morning and night, breastfeeding was primarily a crutch to comfort her, to calm her, to get her to sleep and back to sleep. Of course that meant I was the only one who could do those things, but by then, that ship had long since sailed.

One cool day in early spring, when my daughter was only a few months old, I had another eye-opening encounter, this time at my pediatrician's office. As my daughter and I sat in the waiting room reading *Goodnight Moon,* another mother came in wearing her small baby in a sling on her chest. She looked tired and pale. When her baby started to fuss, she pulled out a bottle, sheepishly. And then she turned to me—a total stranger—to explain why she was bottle-feeding her baby. It was a long story that started with an emergency premature birth and ended with her inability to produce enough milk—what medical professionals delicately call "lactation failure." When the baby showed signs of dehydration, the pediatrician insisted she use formula. About halfway through, she started crying; by the end, she was sobbing. I tried to say comforting, sympathetic things—about how healthy and happy the baby looked, how there's nothing wrong with formula—but it didn't help. She was inconsolable. The most I could do was try to distract my daughter when her insistent little fists started tugging on my shirt. I wasn't about to add to this woman's anguish by breastfeeding right in front of her. I felt guilty enough already. Somehow I'd won a prize that I blithely took for granted but that this woman desperately wanted.

That encounter in my pediatrician's office stayed with me. It was the first time I realized how much shame and despair women can feel when they don't breastfeed. Breastfeeding had been easy for me—not painless and not without frustration, doubt, and embarrassment, but never truly difficult. And because I was lucky, I had escaped the moralizing lectures and public shaming that many nonbreastfeeding mothers endure. Whether or not I was a true believer, I was "in"—beyond reproach, a good mother. My baby didn't sleep through the night, I was working full-time, and we didn't always read to her before bed. But at least I was breastfeeding!

A few years later, after I had stopped breastfeeding my daughter, I had to let go of that slim sense of accomplishment when I came across Hanna Rosin's article about breastfeeding in *The Atlantic*. Rosin was breastfeeding her third child and growing a little fed up with the whole routine. One night she sat down to read the latest scientific and medical research on breastfeeding—something I had never thought to do—and was shocked to discover that "the actual health benefits of breastfeeding are surprisingly thin." The evidence for many of the most hyped benefits, like improving cognitive development, seemed mostly mixed and inconclusive, or the effects were modest. Rosin's article shocked a lot of people, many of whom rushed to attack and dismiss her. But I found her article compelling. If she was even partly right, the zealotry surrounding breastfeeding was even more mystifying than I'd thought.

The final straw came a few months later when I happened to discover how WIC promotes breastfeeding. I was telling a graduate student in my department about my encounter with the anguished woman in the pediatrician's waiting room and wondering aloud about the emotional freight attached to breastfeeding. My graduate student, Emily, a new mother herself, chimed in immediately. "Yeah, what really surprised me is how WIC gives breastfeeding and nonbreastfeeding mothers different benefits." At first, I thought I had misheard. But I hadn't. As a graduate student whose partner was unemployed, Emily's family qualified for the WIC supplemental food program when their baby was born. And because her partner was breastfeeding, she was eligible for all of the perks WIC offers breastfeeding mothers, including qualifying for benefits for twice as long as nonbreastfeeding mothers and receiving better food options.

Until that moment, I had assumed that the breastfeeding imperative was pernicious mostly because it made mothers who don't breastfeed feel guilty. I didn't think they should be made to feel guilty, nor did I think mothers like me, who did breastfeed, had any right to feel smug. Still, I shrugged off those bad dynamics as an unavoidable aspect of parenting, another example of the so-called mommy wars—the vicious disagreements parents sometimes have about child rearing.

But if the US government was effectively punishing poor mothers who didn't breastfeed, *and their babies too*, then the stakes were much higher than I had imagined. And if Rosin was right in saying that there wasn't much benefit to breastfeeding after all, then the government's punitive approach to women who don't breastfeed was shocking.

FOR ME, COMING TO UNDERSTAND the origins and impact of the breastfeeding imperative over the past few years has been disorienting, and sometimes even painful. As a new mother, I desperately wanted to make sure my babies would be healthy and secure. In a world of uncertainty about how to parent and protect our children, most of us are eager to cling to something solid and uncontroversial. Breastfeeding seemed to be just that: proven by science and endorsed by pediatricians, childhood development specialists, and highly respected government agencies and policy organizations around the world. Plus, I was good at it, and so were my babies. I didn't really want to see another side.

But, as time went on, the other side became impossible to ignore. As I was writing this book, people asked me incredulously, "But how could you be *against* breastfeeding?" They knew I was breastfeeding even as I was writing it, and breastfeeding was so good, and wholesome, and pure. . . .

And that's just it. I am not against breastfeeding. I am against *lactivism*. I am against using the particular infant-feeding practices of one privileged demographic to measure people who lack the resources to breastfeed—or simply prefer not to. I am against using a selective reading of medical literature to justify a public health issue. I am against using that public health issue to compel women to breastfeed and to punish those who don't. And I am against government policies that create the expectation that women should comply with the moral imperative to breastfeed by pumping breast milk at work. I am also wary of how the practice of breastfeeding has been quietly but effectively redefined as the consumption of human milk, and with the transformation of breast milk into a highly sought-after commodity that routinely sells on the open market. And I am deeply concerned about lactivist initiatives that treat breast-feeding as an end rather than a means, overlooking, and even neglecting, the needs and interests, and even the lives, of mothers and children.

Through interviews with doctors, policy makers, breastfeeding advocates, La Leche League, WIC recipients, and mothers, this book offers a heartfelt attempt to figure out what's going on with breastfeeding policies and politics in the US, and how we got here. It is also a critique. This is not where, or who, we want to be.

CHAPTER 1

Turning the Tide

I still remember the first time I saw someone breastfeeding. My friend Kim was propped up in her hospital bed with her new baby, just one day old. The baby was latched firmly to one breast, eating hungrily, and my friend was cupping a cabbage leaf over the other breast to relieve the heat and pain of engorgement. The room reeked of cooked cabbage. Kim was a study in incredulity. *"Can you believe this?!"* She had never seen anyone breastfeeding either, and she had never imagined it would involve cabbage leaves. We were both twenty-seven years old, and breastfeeding was as alien as the moon.

As far as world history goes, my friend and I were outliers. Until the beginning of the twentieth century, most women breastfed their babies. As early as 3000 BC, the "lactating goddesses" Ishtar of Babylon and Isis of Egypt were routinely called on to ensure a plentiful supply of milk. The many clay sculptures of these goddesses unearthed throughout the Middle East have led archaeologists to conclude that breastfeeding was held in high regard. The Papyrus Ebers, a medical text written in 1500

BC, includes breastfeeding advice, and there are also references to breastfeeding from the Ptolemaic period. The Indian medical text Susruta Samhita (200 BC) includes specific instructions to start breastfeeding on the fifth day after birth. Hippocrates (460–370 BC), the father of modern medicine, wrote briefly about breastfeeding, and the prolific Greek physician Soranus of Ephesus (200 AD) wrote a medical treatise that included twenty-three chapters on mothering, infant feeding, teething, and childhood illnesses. In Peru, archaeologists have also found clay sculptures of breastfeeding women and their babies that the ancient Peruvian Moche people made as early as 1 AD.

In short, there has never been a time when women didn't breastfeed. But, perhaps more surprising, there has also never been a time when *all* women breastfed. The conventional wisdom these days, at least among lactivists, is that only a small number of women are unable to produce milk. Yet the historical record suggests otherwise. From the ancients on, there have been no shortage of remedies for so-called lactation failure. The Papyrus Ebers recommends rubbing the back of the "failing" mother with oil and warmed swordfish bones. If the swordfish bones didn't work, they called for a wet nurse. The Code of Hammurabi, a Babylonian legal code written around 1700 BC, includes laws regulating wet nursing.

Breastfeeding and wet nurses feature prominently in the Bible too, most famously in Exodus 2:9, when Pharaoh's daughter hired a woman to feed Moses after she rescued him from the bulrushes: "And Pharaoh's daughter said unto her, Take this child away, and nurse it for me, and I will give thee thy wages." Ancient texts from Greece, Rome, and Egypt also make clear that wet nursing was a respectable and well-organized profession regulated by formal contracts.

Less frequently, bottles were also used as an alternative to breastfeeding. In the Egyptian Museum of Antiquities in Cairo there is a nursing flask that dates back to the Alexandrian period. Terra-cotta feeding bottles from circa 1500 BC also attest to the historical use of breastfeeding alternatives, although there is no written record of what those bottles might have contained.

Ancient documents also show that necessity—whether in the form of so-called lactation failure or maternal death—was not the only reason wet nurses were hired. As early as 950 BC, high-status women in Greece employed wet nurses to feed their babies. Privilege has always played a crucial role. In the Ptolemaic period, women used slaves to nurse their babies. From at least the 1200s, royal families throughout Europe employed wet nurses to maintain the fertility of the royal mother. Aristocratic families eventually followed their lead. By the 1880s, hiring a wet nurse was a common practice among families who could afford it. Jane Austen's mother, Cassandra, for example, dispatched each of her eight babies to be wet-nursed in a nearby village. They returned home at eighteen months.

In the United States, by contrast, wet nursing was far less common. During the American colonial period, women generally nursed their babies at least through the second summer of their lives. By the middle of the 1800s, daguerreotype portraits of mothers breastfeeding, sometimes posed with a fair bit of breast exposed, circulated among loved ones as cherished keepsakes. In her book *Mansions of Happiness*, the historian Jill Lepore suggests that husbands might have kept these precious portraits in their breast pockets. In the antiaristocratic atmosphere of the early nation, breastfeeding your own child was a badge of honor—the mark of good mothering and good morals. My great-grandmother, a homesteading cattle rancher who traveled by covered wagon from Texas to Iowa, breastfed my grandmother until she was about two.

By the 1860s or so, mothers found a new option for feeding their babies. Women who didn't breastfeed, for one reason or another, could still hire a wet nurse, as generations of women before them had done. Or they could concoct a homemade formula, combining specific ratios of cow's milk, cream, water, and honey. The world's first commercially available infant formula was invented in 1867, when Henri Nestlé, a pharmacist, allegedly saved the life of a neighbor's child by combining cow's milk with wheat flour and sugar. On the basis of that recipe, he went on to found the Nestlé Company in Vevey, Switzerland. Now a global corporation whose products range from formula to chocolate milk, coffee, and candy, Nestlé's headquarters remain in Vevey to this day.

Finally, in the last two decades of the nineteenth century, as Lepore has shown, breastfeeding rates in America too started to break down along class lines—as had long been the case in Europe. At that point, breastfeeding began to be seen as inappropriate for polite upper-class women. Whereas working-class mothers continued, most often, to breastfeed their babies, wealthier mothers turned increasingly to wet nurses and formula. A Boston study from the early 1900s shows how stark that demographic divide was: while 90 percent of working-class women breastfed their babies, only 17 percent of middle- or upper-class women did so. As Lepore also mentions, one of the striking features of breastfeeding history is that this long-standing demographic trend has now been almost completely reversed. These days breastfeeding is most common among the upper and middle classes while working-class and poor women are more likely to use formula—a practice that has made them vulnerable not only to widespread criticism but, in some cases, punishment.

For most of the twentieth century, as breast-milk substitutes improved and became more widely available, breastfeeding rates plummeted across the social spectrum. In 1912, only 39 percent of Chicago mothers exclusively breastfed their infants. In the 1920s, homemade recipes were improved by adding orange juice or cod liver oil to a baby's diet to reduce a baby's risk of scurvy and rickets. The range of choices seemed to improve again in the next two decades after evaporated milk became widely available at low prices. By the 1950s, more than half of all babies in the United States were fed evaporated milk formula.

When I was born in 1965, my mother did not consider breastfeeding, even for a second. None of her friends breastfed their children, and she thought of it as backward, even faintly repulsive. Her doctor gave her an injection to dry up her milk and recommended formula. When it turned out I was allergic to standard formula, I was switched to a soy-based alternative. Nursing was never an option.

Back then, formula feeding was part of a broader philosophy called "scientific motherhood." Scientific motherhood included hospitalized, doctor supervised, and medicated childbirth and feeding a baby on a strictly prescribed four-hour schedule. Doctors favored formula feeding not least because mothers could measure exactly how much their babies ate, part of a broader trend toward quantification. They often instructed mothers to weigh their babies before and after feedings to monitor their intake. For most midcentury Americans, formula feeding seemed modern, up-to-date, and even sophisticated. It was also socially liberating, offering ordinary mothers a degree of freedom that had been previously accessible only to the upper classes.

STILL, NOT ALL WOMEN EMBRACED that newfound freedom. Small pockets of resistance persisted or emerged across the country. If lactivism has an origin story, its protagonists are the seven Catholic housewives who founded La Leche League in 1956. Mary White and Marian Tompson were breastfeeding their babies together at a Christian Family Movement picnic in the summer of 1956 when they came up with the idea of starting a group to support breastfeeding and "natural" mothering. Along with five other like-minded mothers, they met first at the home of White in Franklin Park, Illinois. Together, they defined a shared mission: to provide support, encouragement, and information to new mothers who were interested in breastfeeding and natural childbirth. They named their new organization after a statue in St. Augustine, Florida, called Nuestra Señora de La Leche y Buen Parto—Our Lady of Plentiful Milk and Good Delivery. Those seven La Leche founders drew on an impressive reserve of collective experience. Between them, they had fifty-six children.

La Leche's core mission was breastfeeding advocacy, but its support for nursing was part of a broader rejection of scientific mothering. La Leche's goal was to return mothering to mothers and to replace the role of the pediatrician as expert with a supportive community of other mothers. Against the cold clinical philosophy of scientific motherhood that placed women at the mercy of doctors, the League urged "naturalism" as a form of empowerment that would let mothers take control of their bodies and their families and embrace their natural bodily functions, first and foremost by breastfeeding. La Leche League was clearly an outlier in an otherwise formula-happy era, but it still managed to grow at an impressively steady rate. From that initial meeting of seven friends in 1956, the League expanded to 43 groups in 1961, 430 in 1966, 1,260 in 1971, and to about 3,000 by 1976.

Historians have argued that La Leche League caught on because it embraced many of the principles that galvanized a newly resurgent feminist movement. The League's focus on what was natural, along with its general suspicion of the medical establishment, resonated with that era's countercultural zeitgeist. In 1971, when the feminist Boston Women's Health Collective published the first mimeographed and stapled edition of *Women and Their Bodies*, one of the most influential and comprehensive feminist critiques of the medical establishment to date, it seemed that La Leche League and modern feminism were roughly on the same page.

Collaboratively written by twelve feminist activists and sold informally as a pamphlet for two years, *Women and Their Bodies* was so popular that it was eventually bought by Simon and Schuster and republished as *Our Bodies, Ourselves* in 1973. Still widely revered as a feminist classic—the most recent edition was published in 2011—*Our Bodies, Ourselves* covers a wide range of issues, including birth control, abortion, childbirth, sexual health, sexual orientation, menopause, gender identity, and mental health.

Like the La Leche mothers, the authors of *Our Bodies, Ourselves* were determined to wrest control of women's bodies from medical experts. Nancy Miriam Hawley, the activist who organized the group, explained years later that they got together because they were fed up with being lectured at and dictated to by male physicians. "We weren't encouraged to ask questions, but to depend on the so-called experts. Not having a say in our own healthcare frustrated and angered us. We didn't have the information we needed, so we decided to find it on our own."

The book pointedly treats women's health as a political and social issue rather than a strictly medical one. But for twenty-first-century readers, who occupy a world in which breastfeeding is highly visible, the fact that *Our Bodies, Ourselves* says almost nothing about breastfeeding is striking. It simply recommends calling La Leche League if "your doctor is not helpful with nursing problems."

The wave of feminism that produced *Our Bodies, Ourselves* was ignited by the publication of another book—Betty Friedan's 1963 runaway best-seller *The Feminine Mystique*. Friedan argued that the grueling monotony of housework and child rearing had produced tracts of depressed suburban wives with squandered lives: a generation of women left wondering, *Is this all?*

There is no evidence that the founders of La Leche League were depressed, but in every other sense they epitomized everything Betty Friedan railed against. They lived in a small Chicago suburb. They believed women should have lots of children—White alone had eleven—and that a woman's place was in the home, taking care of her family. They also believed that the well-being of babies depended first and foremost on maternal attachment and attention. Mothers were not only warned against relying on bottles, they were also advised to avoid other modern conveniences that could be used as "mother substitutes," such as pacifiers, high chairs, baby carriages, and playpens. From the League's perspective, good mothering was a full-time occupation. Mothers were discouraged from working outside the home and encouraged to rank child care above housework and appearances. In an era when women devoured *Better Homes and Gardens* and prided themselves on a well-kept home, League mothers boasted that their messy homes showed that they valued "people over things."

For a while, at least, the League's philosophies suggested a countercultural orientation that put them at odds with mainstream America. But the group was also deeply conservative from the outset—light years away from the hippie and feminist organizations with which it seemed, at least initially, to align. The gulf between the feminist movement and La Leche League grew most visible as the debate over abortion heated up in the years before the landmark *Roe v. Wade* Supreme Court decision legalizing abortion in 1973. Using slogans like "the personal is political," second-wave feminists made issues like abortion and reproductive rights central to their platform. They believed that the first step toward the liberation of women was the liberation of their bodies, and the focus of their efforts was a woman's right to choose.

In 1971, as abortion began to take center stage as one of the most pressing and polarizing issues in American politics, La Leche was riven by internal disagreement. As Catholics, all of the leaders were staunch opponents of abortion, but they disagreed over whether La Leche should take an official pro-life stance or remain silent. White strongly believed they needed to go public. "I think we're being two-faced to say we want to help mothers and babies, but at the same time, by our silence, to condone killing these little ones. To 'not take a stand' is taking a stand. It says we don't care. I think we should care." Some of the founding mothers agreed with her. Others, however, believed La Leche should avoid the controversy surrounding abortion.

When the issue came to a vote, the founding mothers were split four against three, and those who favored taking a stance against abortion lost. Undeterred, they took their battle public a few months later at the 1971 La Leche League convention in Chicago, where White pleaded for La Leche League "to take a stand in support of all mothers and their unborn babies." Although she received a standing ovation, the board subsequently passed a motion "stating that any LLL member who brought up the subject of abortion at an LLL function would summarily be dismissed from La Leche League."

La Leche also took a principled and very vocal stand against women working outside the home. The first loose-leaf copy of the League's publication *The Womanly Art of Breastfeeding*, published in 1958, explicitly instructed mothers to stay home with their children. League members did not work, and the League only allowed full-time mothers to be group leaders. Even the revised 1981 edition of the League's manual strongly encouraged stay-at-home mothering: "Our plea to any mother who is thinking about taking an outside job is 'if at all possible, don't.'"

By the early 1980s, however, that antiwork position had started to affect the League's membership. In 1975, 31 percent of mothers with infants less than one year old were in the paid labor force. By 1980 it was 39 percent, and in 1987 52 percent of mothers with infants under one year of age were employed outside the home. As membership and organization funding faltered, the League's leaders made a strategic decision to relax the organization's opposition to working mothers and to retool its mission to address the hurdles confronting mothers who were trying to combine working and breastfeeding. Meetings and publications started to cover such topics as "How do I prepare my infant for daycare?" "What should I look for in a pump?" and "What is the easiest way to wean a baby?" Still, even through the mid-1990s, the organization's literature continued to make clear that stay-at-home mothering was the ideal. To this day, the majority of women you might meet at La Leche meetings are stay-at-home mothers.

FOR ITS FIRST FIFTEEN YEARS, La Leche League was decidedly marginal, a breastfeeding advocacy organization that presided over a steady decline in the number of American women who breastfed. In 1956, 32 percent of American women initiated breastfeeding. In 1971, the nadir of American breastfeeding, only 24 percent of women initiated breastfeeding, and only 5 percent were still breastfeeding at six months.

The reasons are not hard to fathom. Mothers were also entering the workplace in increasing numbers. Perhaps even more importantly, formula was considered a safe and healthy alternative to breastfeeding, and most doctors recommended it. There was very little research on the potential benefits of breastfeeding (that would not start until later in the 1970s), and most doctors were so committed to formula feeding they had no idea how to support a mother who wanted to breastfeed.

One mother who experienced that lack of support firsthand was Edith White. I tracked White down because she was an early convert to the breastfeeding cause who, years later, grew disillusioned with advocacy practices that elevated breastfeeding above the health and lives of children. I caught up with her just as she was embarking on a long cross-country drive from Arizona to Oregon.

When Edith White married Don Tibbetts in 1965, she was young and idealistic and determined to be a good wife. She followed her new husband from Massachusetts to graduate school at the University of Illinois at Champaign-Urbana and supported them both by teaching second grade.

When their first baby, Andrew, was born in 1968, White assumed she would breastfeed. Among her family and friends in Boston, breastfeeding was still common practice. But far away from home, she relied on the advice of her doctors, whom she describes, in retrospect, as clueless. "I had what I now look back on as a typical experience of my generation trying to breastfeed my first child—a healthy, full-term, normal baby. The advice I received from my two male doctors was completely counterproductive. The obstetrician put me on high-dose birth control pills, which were not good for your milk supply in terms of your physiology, and then my pediatrician told me I had to breastfeed on a four-hour schedule." We know now that both estrogen-based birth control pills and a strict four-hour feeding schedule are likely to inhibit full milk production. Two months later White gave up in frustration. Her baby fussed and screamed at her breast, and she worried that her milk supply was too low. "It just wasn't working."

By 1971, the family had moved to Philadelphia, and White was pregnant with her second child, Christopher. Despite the disappointment of her first efforts, she remained committed to the idea of breastfeeding. This time, however, she ventured beyond the doctor's office to an organization called Childbirth Education and Nursing Mothers of Greater Philadelphia, which held birth and breastfeeding classes. "I learned, then, for the first time, how breastfeeding was supposed to work. I learned that it was frequent feeding that kept the milk supply up." Attending classes and talking to nursing mothers made White realize she had gotten bad advice from her male doctors. Their ignorance had caused her to fail at breastfeeding her first child. Once she connected with ordinary mothers, however, everything changed: "After one half-hour meeting, they basically told me what I needed to know!" White went on to successfully breastfeed her second son for eighteen months and did not return to teaching.

Instead, she was so impressed with Nursing Mothers that she started to volunteer for them and eventually trained to be a breastfeeding advocate. She told me she was drawn to Nursing Mothers because it shared La Leche's commitment to breast-feeding advocacy, without its religious and moral conservatism.

"You know, with La Leche, all the founders were Catholic, glorified having eleven children, or seven children, having the baby in bed with you, nursing constantly, sort of opposed to birth control. Nursing Mothers was much more liberal. So I felt compatible with them. And I went through the training, which is about helping new mothers, answering her questions, giving her moral support." Gradually, White rose through the ranks of the organization. She became a regional advisor, and she was steeped in what she now calls the "breastfeeding philosophy." By the time her daughter, Amy, was born in 1974, White was such a true believer that she breastfed her for two and a half years. In contemporary terms, she had become a committed lactivist—a person who firmly believed breastfeeding was the best choice for everyone.

White's conversion to lactivism followed a typical path for women of her generation. Her initial failure with breastfeeding triggered a personal crisis. She was frustrated that her doctors had been unable to help her figure out how to breastfeed her first child, and the difference between the experience she had with her first and second child made her appreciate how important an organization like Nursing Mothers could be. Without these grassroots peer communities, women's only source of information would be doctors, most of whom were men. She threw herself into the cause with the conviction that women needed to assert more control over their own health care.

As it happened, White entered the world of breastfeeding advocacy just as it was making headlines and mobilizing
women and men around the world. In 1970, 11 million babies
died each year before their first birthday. Most of those deaths
were in Africa and Southeast Asia, where, on average, almost
130 out of every 1,000 died every year. In India alone, 2.6 million babies died in 1970.

That year, 1970, was also the first year it was possible to access reliable data on infant mortality for most of the world. The
horrific statistics that emerged quickly became news headlines,
capturing the attention of world health officials, government
leaders, international institutions, and concerned citizens the
world over. Journalists who traveled to the poorest countries
translated the staggering number of infant deaths—*eleven million in one year*—into heartbreaking stories and images of sick
and suffering babies with enormous eyes, distended bellies, and
shriveled limbs. At the time, 11 million people was more than
the populations of New York and Los Angeles combined. It was
a massacre.

Of course there were many reasons that eleven million babies were dying every year. In the Soviet Union, most infants
died of pneumonia and other respiratory infections. Malaria,
measles, injury, and sudden infant death syndrome (SIDS) also
caused many infant deaths. But in Africa and Southeast Asia,
those regions of the world that had the highest infant mortality
rates, malnutrition and diarrhea were by far the leading causes
of infant mortality.

Once the world began to pay attention, the link between
formula feeding and babies dying of malnutrition and diarrhea
was not hard to draw. In the 1960s and 1970s, many developing
countries were going through the process social scientists call

"modernization." Parents were leaving their families and villages to look for work in the city. Often they left young children behind with their grandparents. Or they brought the children along and left them with caregivers while they worked. In the cities, they were introduced to new ideas and styles that would identify them as modern—and baby formula was prominent among them.

Formula companies were quick to see that the dramatic and widespread social changes taking place in the developing world opened a large potential market for formula. Nestlé expanded by leaps and bounds to capture the international market, building factories in developing countries and opening sales centers all over the world. In 1981, the world market for formula was estimated at $2 billion. Nestlé commanded a 50 percent share of that market, and the other 50 percent was divided among three American companies: Abbott Laboratories, Bristol-Myers, and American Home Products.

Nestlé in particular moved into these new markets aggressively and on numerous fronts. Print and radio ads touting the health benefits of formula were everywhere, or close to it. In Brazil, formula was the third-most commonly advertised product, after cigarettes and soap. Nestlé also began the now-familiar strategy of offering new and expecting mothers incentivizing giveaways. The World Health Organization (WHO) estimated that about five million free baby bottles were distributed each year in India, Nigeria, Ethiopia, and the Philippines. The average clinic in Nigeria received as many as eight thousand free cans of formula per year. In 1975 Ross Laboratories clarified the logic of formula freebies in an internal selling manual: "When one considers that for every 100 infants discharged from the hospital on a particular formula brand, approximately

93 infants will remain on that brand, the importance of hospital selling becomes obvious."

This same logic informed what eventually emerged as one of Nestlé's most outrageous marketing tactics—the so-called Nestlé nurses. In the 1970s, formula companies routinely employed women to visit new mothers in hospital maternity wards and at home to offer advice on feeding and caring for their new babies. Nestlé often dressed their salespeople in starched white nurses' uniforms, complete with the wimple-like veils traditionally worn by nuns. As they helped mothers cope with newborn babies, these Nestlé nurses promoted their company's formula, conveying the false impression that they were independent health-care professionals rather than formula company employees.

There are no hard figures with which to measure the effects of formula marketing on formula feeding or to correlate formula feeding with the rise in infant mortality. But health officials nonetheless agree that there was a "marked jump in the rate of gastroenteritis and malnutrition relating to the improper use of infant formula and the associated feeding equipment, such as bottles and nipples" in the 1960s and 1970s. In a 1981 *New York Times* article, the director general of WHO estimated that "infants breastfed less than six months, or not at all, have a mortality rate 5–10 times higher in the second six months of life than those breastfed six months or more."

The underlying reasons for these deaths were well documented. First of all, formula comes in powder form and must be mixed with clean water. Poor mothers in developing countries often lack access to clean water or the means to boil water. In the absence of ready access to clean water, they resorted to contaminated water from rivers, lakes, streams, ponds or urban taps. That contaminated water was not only mixed with powdered formula, it was also used to clean bottles. In 1979, researchers in Indonesia found "gross contamination" in baby bottles from fecal organisms in the water supply and concluded that babies fed from a bottle should be classified "high risk."

Another problem was cost. Mothers who tried free formula risked losing their own milk supply and becoming dependent on formula, which they subsequently had to pay for themselves. That formula was shockingly expensive. It could consume 30 to 50 percent of a poor family's income. Poor mothers often attempted to defray that crippling cost by diluting formula in an effort to make each can last longer. One study conducted in Indonesia in 1979 found that only one in four mothers mixed the formula reasonably close to its recommended strength. A doctor in Bangladesh explained that babies were often fed "milk" that was little more than white water. A Jamaican mother who brought her starving twins into a clinic explained that one can of formula lasted the two children two weeks. It should have lasted two days.

Mothers also tried to save money by storing unfinished formula. One nurse who worked with Peruvian Indians in the Amazon explained that when infants didn't finish a bottle, mothers saved it until the next feeding. "Stored at room temperature, in a tropical country, you have explosive bacterial growth. So the bottle becomes a lethal instrument."

The link between infant mortality and formula feeding was first publicized in a British magazine called *The New Internationalist*, in 1973. "The Baby Food Tragedy" was a searing account of how formula feeding led to malnutrition, diarrhea, and death in poor countries where people had no access to clean drinking water, couldn't read instructions, and were too poor to buy enough formula.

Nestlé responded to the article by inviting journalists and activists to its headquarters in Switzerland, in an effort to explain Nestlé's approach to infant nutrition. That turned out to be a big mistake. Mike Muller, from the British NGO War on Want, accepted the invitation and then went on to publish an exposé of the formula industry called *The Baby Killer*. Whereas Nestlé had tried to pass off its third-world sales efforts as genuine concern for infant health, Muller saw only a cynical profit grab. His pamphlet went beyond the claim that formula was killing babies in poor countries to accuse formula companies of responsibility for those deaths by driving the growing demand for formula through aggressive "commercial promotion."

Muller's pamphlet was initially published in English and sold by War on Want for thirty-five pence a copy. It ultimately gained much greater visibility, however, after the publication of the German translation. Renamed *Nestlé Kills Babies*, the translation prompted Nestlé to sue for libel. In the course of building their defense, the pamphlet's authors collected reports, medical studies, affidavits, and eyewitness accounts from the developing world—documents that would eventually form the wellspring of the subsequent and continuing campaign against baby formula marketing.

That campaign was next taken up in 1976 when a religious order in the United States called Sisters of the Precious Blood sued Bristol-Myers for unethical marketing practices in developing countries. An out-of-court settlement required Bristol-Myers to acknowledge its marketing practices. Then in 1977, the American NGO Infant Formula Action Coalition (INFACT) launched the Nestlé boycott, which quickly spread to Canada, Australia, and New Zealand. The boycott's main goal was to limit the company's marketing reach by eliminating direct marketing to consumers, eliminating freebies and handouts, and stopping the practice of dressing salespeople as medical professionals. The campaign called for consumers to boycott all Nestlé products until it complied with these demands. In the annals of modern breastfeeding, the Nestlé boycott is a major landmark.

White recalls how the Nestlé boycott also fanned the flames of breastfeeding advocacy back home. Americans' growing awareness of Nestlé's reckless and cynical promotion of formula in the developing world made them more sympathetic to breastfeeding in general. When Nursing Mothers of Greater Philadelphia publicized information about the formula companies and the boycott, White remembers that "of course it was a slam dunk! Of course we believed that what the formula companies are doing is wrong, and of course when we go to the grocery store we're going to check labels to make sure we're not buying Nestlé products!" Even though Nursing Mothers was focused on community advocacy at the local level, its members increasingly felt they were part of something bigger. As a perfect example of the need to "think globally, act locally," which was such a clarion call of left politics in that era, breastfeeding advocacy acquired new relevance and visibility.

Meanwhile in the United States, La Leche League was growing by leaps and bounds, including several chapters outside the US. Other breastfeeding advocacy groups, like Nursing Mothers, were also proliferating in communities across the country. And, for the first time ever, American breastfeeding initiation rates started to go up—from 24 percent in 1971 to 33 percent in 1975, to a stunning 54 percent by 1980. Public interest and debate around breastfeeding, combined with new sources of community support for breastfeeding mothers, were having an impact, edging breastfeeding back from the margins to the mainstream of American parenting.

Breastfeeding's new prominence also had an unanticipated effect on the Special Supplemental Nutrition Program for Women, Infants, and Children (WIC). WIC was inaugurated in 1974 by the US Department of Agriculture in an effort to provide food for at-risk families. From its inception, WIC counselors were instructed to encourage women to breastfeed. According to White, they seemed, however, woefully ill equipped to do that. White describes the first generation of WIC counselors as young, middle-class, white women with degrees in nutrition. "Typically they were in their twenties, fresh out of college. They understand all the wonderful benefits of breastfeeding and are very gung ho." But when they came into contact with WIC clients, they were often out of their depth. "The client might be a woman pregnant with her fifth child, and here's this twenty-four-year-old nutritionist who is supposed to tell her what children should eat and how to breastfeed." WIC counselors had very little life experience, and almost no idea of how to support breastfeeding. Few of them had children, and even fewer had breastfed. What they did have were instructions to encourage their clients to breastfeed and money to spend on training them.

In the Philadelphia area, WIC counselors started to ask White's organization, Nursing Mothers, to provide breastfeeding counseling and advocacy training. Nursing Mothers didn't have the resources to respond to all those requests, but White and a friend started to take on those training sessions as independent contractors, and eventually they started a company. For about twenty years, from roughly 1976 to 1996, White and her partner ran a business teaching breastfeeding classes to counselors working for WIC. She estimates they taught breast-feeding techniques and troubleshooting tactics to about ten thousand WIC employees across the country.

The growing demand for breastfeeding information and advice that White was experiencing at the local level was matched by expanding interest at the national and international levels. In 1976, German filmmaker Peter Krieg released a small independent film called *Bottle Babies*, about formula-fed babies dying of malnutrition in Kenya. Another milestone in American breastfeeding advocacy occurred in 1978, when Edward Kennedy, the Democratic senator from Massachusetts, convened a Senate hearing on baby food marketing. The televised Kennedy hearings brought heart-wrenching testimony from doctors and nurses in developing countries into living rooms across the country. Americans looked on as persistent questioning by Senator Kennedy prompted a reluctant Nestlé executive to concede that formula should not be used where mothers lack access to clean water.

Kennedy's Senate hearing played an important role in raising the profile of the Nestlé boycott domestically and prompting international health organizations to take action against the dangers of formula feeding. One year later, in 1979, WHO and UNICEF convened a conference to consider a marketing code that would specify what companies could and couldn't do to promote and sell baby formula. A number of the conference participants banded together to form the International Baby Food Action Network, the organization that drafted the marketing code, campaigned for its implementation, and assumed responsibility for monitoring the baby food industry's compliance with it. In 1981 the World Health Assembly adopted the

International Code of Marketing of Breast-Milk Substitutes. That code banned direct advertising of baby formula to consumers; the distribution of freebies such as formula, bottles, company pens, and prescription pads; and the practice of misrepresenting salespeople as medical professionals. Only the United States voted against it.

The marketing code and the boycott have dogged Nestlé ever since. After three years of continued resistance, Nestlé capitulated in 1984 to continuing and increasing pressure from activists and world health organizations by agreeing to implement the code in developing countries. At that point, six years after it started, the Nestlé boycott was suspended. But the suspension was short lived. Four years later, when monitors discovered that formula companies continued to violate provisions of the code, the Nestlé boycott resumed. Amazingly, it has been in place ever since—according to Anwar Fazal, the longest and most extensive consumer boycott in history.

Activism surrounding breastfeeding and the Nestlé boycott elevated the status of breastfeeding among international health organizations. Beginning in the early 1980s, WHO and UNICEF began to push breastfeeding as a key strategy in their arsenal against infant mortality and childhood disease, and many regional health organizations followed suit. Almost overnight, breastfeeding advocacy became an institutional priority. In 1982, UNICEF launched a major new initiative called the Child Survival and Development Revolution; breastfeeding promotion was one of the four key strategic pillars of its new agenda. In its 1985 annual report, UNICEF described its breastfeeding support strategies in a number of the poorest countries of the world, urging continued vigilance against incursions from formula. In 1984 and 1985, UNICEF even issued pro-breastfeeding postage stamps.

By the mid-1980s, breastfeeding had achieved mainstream status as a top priority of the world's global health organizations. La Leche's many years of advocacy had finally begun to pay off as the tide of public opinion started to swing in favor of breastfeeding. Activism around the Nestlé boycott was clearly the most visible and important milestone in that transition, but that activism was successful in large part because of the social and organizational background, in local breastfeeding support and advocacy groups and networks, that sustained it. Globally, and in the US as well, the tide had turned.

CHAPTER 2

A Consensus Emerges

I n the wake of the Nestlé boycott, breastfeeding acquired a new image. Over the course of ten short years, it had been transformed from an archaic practice that limited women's freedom into an important moral and political activity that protected vulnerable mothers and children against the predatory practices of greedy corporations. It was also a symbol of solidarity in the struggle against world poverty and hunger. Those positive associations have remained more or less intact ever since, and they have been bolstered by a steady stream of research attesting to the many and various health benefits breastfeeding is supposed to offer. At this point, the halo effect of breastfeeding is considerable. Anyone who breastfeeds, as I have, will know exactly what that halo effect means in terms of social acceptance and moral standing.

It's no surprise, then, that breastfeeding rates have climbed steadily since the 1970s, from 24 percent in 1971 to 79 percent in 2014. And it's perhaps no surprise either that breastfeeding has become a consensus issue, a widely accepted practice embraced by Americans of all stripes, across the political spectrum. To be *against* breastfeeding is almost sacrilegious. The few who dare to question its importance, as the journalist Hanna Rosin did in her *Atlantic* article "The Case Against Breast-Feeding," risk being subjected to insults and ridicule.

The truth is that in the United States, breastfeeding has become much more than simply a way to feed a baby. It is a way of showing the world who you are and what you believe in. At least four very different segments of the American population—feminists, fundamentalists, yuppies, and hipsters—have appropriated breastfeeding as a marker of a larger set of values and beliefs. Breastfeeding may not be quite all things to all people, but it is an unexpected number of things to a wide range of people.

FOR THE FIRST GENERATION OF LACTIVISTS who embraced and extolled breastfeeding from the late 1950s on, breastfeeding was a woman's issue, if not exactly a feminist one. La Leche League explicitly emphasized the need for women to take control over their bodies and resist the so-called expertise of male doctors—even if they didn't challenge male authority in general. The founders of La Leche League were practicing Catholics who believed women should stay at home to look after their children, supported by husbands with paid work. But the League's emphasis on a woman's right to choose how to feed her baby made their message roughly compatible with a resurgent feminist movement that was focused on expanding women's rights on many different fronts.

Scholars tend to organize the history of feminism into waves. Beginning in the 1800s and early 1900s, so-called first-wave feminists like the suffragettes fought for women's right to vote, to hold elected office, to inherit and own property, and to enjoy full rights in citizenship. They also fought for access to higher education, employment in sectors normally reserved for men, the right to seek divorce, and better pay. They were focused primarily on showing that women deserved the same rights as men because they were equal to men in terms of their abilities and skills.

The second wave was triggered by the 1963 publication of Betty Friedan's book *The Feminine Mystique*. Women, she argued, were depressed because they were financially, mentally, physically, and intellectually subservient to men. The role of idealized housewife forced women into small lives and squandered their potential. Friedan was describing the experiences of herself and her fellow graduates from the Smith College class of 1942. Born in Peoria, Illinois, Friedan graduated from Smith with a degree in psychology and went to work as a journalist for leftist and trade union publications. In 1947 she married Carl Friedan and, while pregnant with their second child, was fired from her position as staff writer at the *UE News*, the trade paper of the the United Electrical, Radio, and Machine Workers. Living in suburban New York, she stayed home with their children and worked as a freelance writer, evidently not very happily.

Friedan was concerned primarily with equality in the workplace. For her and for many other women of her generation, women's liberation meant, first and foremost, financial independence and a fulfilling career outside the home. And, as the record shows, second-wave feminism instigated an increase of women in the workforce, as legions of women migrated out of the house and into the working world. Over the past five decades, through the efforts of these second-wave feminists, women have come closer to achieving salary parity with men, have gained respect, and have achieved increasing levels of authority by rising through the ranks of corporations, hospitals, universities, and government. Even if much still remains to be done, thanks to second-wave feminists, women have broken through many glass ceilings.

But second-wave feminism was not only about parity in the workplace. Betty Friedan spent much of her public life locked in a notorious rivalry with Gloria Steinem, based on a profound disagreement over what issues feminists should take up and which direction the feminist movement should take.

Steinem grew up in Toledo, Ohio, and graduated from Smith about fifteen years after Friedan. Steinem, too, became a journalist, writing freelance articles for magazines like *Esquire* and *Show* and eventually cofounding the feminist *Ms.* magazine. But unlike Friedan, Steinem focused on issues that highlighted the need for women to take control of their bodies, including sexual harassment, domestic violence, and reproductive rights—a term she coined herself. By deftly deploying slogans like "The personal is political," this strand of second-wave feminism was instrumental in legalizing abortion, raising the age of statutory rape, altering the definition of consent in the context of sexual relationships, and limiting the extent to which a woman's sexual history could be used as evidence against her in court.

For these second-wave feminists, women's liberation was a sexual revolution and a declaration of female difference and power. Early in her career as a journalist, Steinem went undercover as a Playboy Bunny at the New York Playboy Club and wrote an exposé about the way bunnies were treated. Other feminists developed powerful critiques of law, liberalism, literature, history, science, and, like the Boston Women's Health Collective, medicine.

The feminist commitment to exposing the power of the patriarchy aligned them with the black power movement, which was also building a critique against a system that was structured against them. Like the black power movement, the women's liberation movement issued a fundamental challenge against the dominance of white male norms. In 1969, Steinem made the connection between the two movements explicit in her instantly famous *New York Magazine* article "After Black Power, Women's Liberation."

As the slogan "Black is beautiful" suggested, equality was not only about being tolerated but *recognized*. For African Americans, one symbol of that difference was the Afro hairstyle. After decades of beauty products designed to straighten the stigmatized curly hair of African Americans and make it as "white" as possible, the Afro was a defiant expression of black pride.

For some feminists, the defiant expression of female pride was breastfeeding. Support for breastfeeding was a component of feminism's focus on sexuality and reproduction. It formed part of the critique of the medicalization of pregnancy, childbirth, and infant feeding—normal life events that women should have more control over. It was also an expression of pride in a bodily function that had been stigmatized. Breastfeeding was something women could uniquely do and something that had been dismissed by male doctors who encouraged mothers to feed their babies formula out of bottles. Like abortion, breastfeeding was an issue that made feminist claims—that the personal is political—seem immediate and compelling.

For many women, breastfeeding continues to be a form of empowerment. It emphasizes the power of women's bodies to nurture and feed another human being. It's an expression of female pride and, often, solidarity. A new generation of mothers, many of whom were raised by ardent feminists with fulfilling careers, has decided against combining work and motherhood. They have chosen to quit their jobs to stay home, parent, and, not least, fulfill the mandate to breastfeed.

But for all the women we hear about who have left the workforce to raise children, many more are still trying to combine working and parenting. The current generation of working women are doing this differently than their mothers. They are trying to force the workplace, and other public spaces, to acknowledge the needs of working mothers and make changes to accommodate them. A woman might, for example, take her infant with her when she attends a meeting at work while she is still on maternity leave. Or her children might come to her office after school, instead of going home to an empty house. A mother might arrange to leave work at 3:45 twice a week to take her daughter to soccer games. These choices are often intended to push back against the assumption or expectation that women can only climb the professional ladder if they behave as if they have no family.

It is this line of feminism that drives current activism around breastfeeding in public. With famous moms like Gisele Bündchen and Gwen Stefani making a point of being photographed breastfeeding, the right to breastfeed in public has gained enormous traction. These women are not exhibitionists, as some critics allege; they are activists who are seizing public space to make a valuable political point about women's rights to feed their babies how, when, and where they choose. *This is what women's lives look like, this is what women do, this is what it takes to raise healthy, happy children. Deal with it, already.*

But what is surprisingly missing from most contemporary feminist discourse is any discussion of a woman's right *not* to breastfeed. Formula feeding is almost never presented as a feminist issue—and those few feminists who have balked at the breastfeeding imperative, including Alissa Quart, Hanna Rosin, and Elisabeth Badinter, remain the exceptions who prove the rule. The language of "choice," which figured so prominently in the struggle of second-wave feminists and still animates debates about abortion and other reproductive rights, is conspicuously absent when we discuss infant feeding.

MANY MIDDLE- AND UPPER-CLASS AMERICANS arrived at their commitment to breastfeeding through a different route: attachment parenting, the most popular and widely practiced contemporary parenting philosophy. In 1992, William Sears and his wife, Martha, published *The Baby Book*. By 2012, *The Baby Book* had been translated into eighteen languages and sold more than 1.5 million copies. As *Time* magazine put it in its provocative 2012 cover article, "Are you Mom Enough?": "If you've had a baby in the 21st century, chances are good that you've encountered *The Baby Book*. Chances are also good that, consciously or not, you've practiced some derivative of attachment parenting or been influenced by its message that mothers and babies evolved to be close to each other." Attachment parents are one of the groups that has elevated breastfeeding beyond mere feeding practice to a core value and commitment symbolic of a broader parenting and lifestyle philosophy.

Attachment parenting is an offshoot of the attachment theory developed by John Bowlby and made famous by the child psychologist Mary Ainsworth. It begins with the idea that normal child and adult development depends on forming a strong emotional bond with caregivers during childhood. Ainsworth devised a well-known psychological experiment called the

Strange Situation to assess the quality of a young child's attachment. A child enters a room with her primary caregiver; a stranger enters the room and interacts with the parent and child; the caregiver leaves the room; the caregiver returns to the room, reuniting with the child. A securely attached child, Ainsworth claimed, would explore the room and toys freely when the parent was present, interact with the stranger when the parent was present, be upset when the parent left the room, and reunite happily with the parent when he returned. Children who did not follow this script were categorized as ambivalent-insecure, avoidant-insecure, or disorganized.

The key to ensuring you don't end up with a child who is insecure or, even worse, disorganized, is attachment parenting. Proper and secure attachment is developed through sensitive, responsive, and emotionally available parenting, and it starts before birth. Parents are encouraged to talk and sing to their baby while she is still in the womb, to massage and play with her through the mother's skin, and to play music for her. Sometimes attachment parents opt to give birth at home, so that the child is born into a more soothing, less clinical environment. At birth, the baby should be placed immediately on the mother's bare chest to initiate skin-to-skin contact so that the baby can be comforted by the familiar sound and rhythm of the mother's heartbeat. The baby should also be brought to the nipple very soon after birth so that she can nurse. If the baby has been born in a hospital, hospital staff are encouraged to delay most of the procedures that are often performed immediately after the baby is born (weighing, measuring, cleaning and suctioning, the heel stick, and the vitamin K injection) or to do them unobtrusively while the baby is nursing or lying on the mother's chest.

But it's not until you get home from the hospital that the real work of attachment parenting begins. The *Time* magazine article on attachment parenting describes the experience in a wonderfully deadpan tone: "Then for months, Beauregard sat on the couch in her Denver-area living room, nursing her infant from sunup to sundown. She nursed much of the night as well, since the baby slept in bed with Beauregard and her husband Daniel."

Although attachment parenting is really more a state of mind—treating your child with respect, paying attention and being responsive to his needs, and being consistently loving, caring, and present—there are also certain inviolable practices that define it, and breastfeeding is at the very top of the list. Breastfeeding is crucial to proper attachment because it offers intimate physical contact that helps mothers and infants bond. Some attachment parenting gurus argue that breastfeeding synchronizes mothers and infants, enabling mothers to understand and respond to their babies' cues more intuitively. These gurus advocate not only nursing but nursing on demand and child-led weaning. Mothers who practice attachment parenting often nurse their children well into toddlerhood.

Attachment parenting also involves a practice called "baby wearing," which means carrying your baby in a sling, nestled against your body, rather than using a stroller. Baby Björn makes a well-known baby carrier, but real attachment parents tend to use slings. Slings are pieces of fabric, preferably organic cotton, that wrap around the body in a range of complicated ways. One friend of mine wore her baby in one all day long—as she made meals in the kitchen, talked on the phone, and vacuumed. Other parents only wear the sling as an alternative to a stroller—outside the house on walks but not necessarily at home all day long. The message that baby wearing is closer to nature is brought home by the fact that many popular slings are decorated in ethnic-looking colors and prints imported from places like the Amazon rain forest or rural Vietnam, places where we imagine attachment parenting is seamlessly integrated into everyday life.

Attachment parenting also involves cosleeping—having a baby sleep in bed with the mother or with both parents. The message here is that parenting is not just a day job. Babies need parenting, security, and comfort around the clock, and that security can best be provided by the warmth and safety of nearby parents, day and night. That intimacy also makes it easier for mothers to perceive and respond to their babies' needs and to feed them on demand, instantly. Ideally, the baby never wakes up alone, never finds herself isolated behind the bars of a crib, and never cries without being heard. As children grow up, parents who practice attachment parenting often have siblings sleep together to further protect them from the trauma of going to sleep or waking up alone.

Much more than a parenting philosophy, attachment parenting is a way of life, both because it demands so much time and focus—and because there's so much at stake. Real attachment parenting requires that one parent, almost always the mother, dedicate herself to parenting full-time to establish and nurture the secure child-parent attachment. Attachment parents do not leave children with a babysitter. I know many mothers who, even by the time their children were five or six years old, had never once left them with a babysitter, not even a grandmother. Others boast that they have never missed putting their child to bed. The parents in the *Time* magazine article explained, with evident pride, "There are no date nights."

We've heard a great deal lately about women with high-powered degrees from Harvard Business School or Yale Law School leaving promising careers to stay at home with their children. Some of these women bring the competitive zeal they brought to graduate school and work into parenting, and they practice attachment parenting because it promises to produce superior children—children who are healthier, smarter, and more secure. This level of commitment to parenting works well for many families, and it does seem likely to have benefits for some children, especially those who require more attention and care.

At the same time, however, it sets up a parenting standard that families who do not have a stay-at-home parent cannot possibly live up to. Those parents often practice some watered-down version of attachment parenting, generally buying into the philosophy but unwilling or unable to commit to the whole enchilada. I call this "half-baked attachment parenting." Half-baked attachment parenting is in fact my own parenting "philosophy." When my daughter and son were babies, I was home for months. I breastfed them a lot, although maybe not always on demand, and when they napped, it was often in my arms or on my lap. I rarely left the house; I never let them cry. I talked to them, I played with them, and I paid attention to them. I still spend part of many nights sleeping with a child. OK, all of most nights.

I also did some things that seem generally in line with attachment parenting but are even a bit more extreme. I opposed pacifiers. I didn't want to silence my baby by sticking a piece of rubber in her mouth. I was also against electric swings, bouncy seats, and walkers: really anything designed to keep babies happy and give parents a break. And I took a very firm stand against baths. We didn't bathe our babies for two or three weeks after they were born because I got it into my head that baths are traumatizing and that our baby should be comforted for as long as possible by the familiar smell of the womb. Talk about half-baked.

But my husband and I also did a lot of things attachment parents would never do. When we brought them home from the hospital, our babies slept in a wooden cradle handed down from my great-grandmother, not in our bed and not even in a crib that would have passed muster with the Consumer Product Safety Commission. We hired babysitters and went out to dinner. Before our daughter turned two, we went to Paris for five days and left her with my mother. We had a stroller, not a sling. I went back to work before my children turned one, mostly by choice, and our children went to day care. Once I concluded that "self-weaning" was not on her agenda, I weaned my daughter when she was two. I didn't wait for my son to self-wean either. And I have *definitely* missed more than one bedtime, sometimes even on purpose.

There have been recent signs of a backlash against attachment parenting for making onerous and unrealistic demands on parents and setting them up for a life of abject servitude or failure. The French philosopher and feminist Elisabeth Badinter's book *The Conflict* makes the case that mothers in particular are held hostage as they sleep with their babies, wear their babies, and nurse their babies around the clock. Blogger and feminist Jessica Valenti's *Why Have Kids?* shows that even stay-at-home moms feel like "bad mothers" when judged by the standards of attachment parenting. Working moms feel even worse, and attachment parenting fuels those infamous "mommy wars" in which working mothers and stay-at-home mothers allegedly compete to establish the superiority of their own method of parenting.

But attachment parenting also fuels a war between middle- and working-class mothers. It sets up a model of good motherhood that only women who can afford to stay at home can ever achieve. Wrapped up in the broader philosophy of attachment parenting, breastfeeding is embraced as a moral imperative that also acts as a strong marker of social status. Women breastfeed in part to maintain that status, and they sometimes use breastfeeding as a way to police its boundaries. A wealthy stay-at-home mom I know once remarked, "If they can't take care of their children," by which she meant stay home with them and breastfeed, "they shouldn't be allowed to have them." As a central plank of the attachment parenting philosophy, the breastfeeding imperative fuels ugly divisions between mothers who can afford to take up mothering as a full-time occupation and mothers who can't.

THE TYPED AND MIMEOGRAPHED PAMPHLET that preceded the publication of *Our Bodies, Ourselves* is still available on the organization's website. Reading it now in the second decade of the twenty-first century is eye-opening precisely because it is so deeply and radically political. This women's health manifesto almost completely ignores medicine and medical research and instead lets the voices and experience of other women speak directly to readers. Topics like reproduction, pregnancy, and childbirth are treated as fundamentally social and political issues, involving rights and legislation rather than breathing exercises or epidurals.

The book's politics and jargon are so casually radical that they seem almost unrecognizable. The first chapter is titled

"Women, Medicine, and Capitalism." It deals with the commodification of female bodies, alienation, subjugation, and the "mystification" performed by medical schools and medical jargon. Not only do the authors call for universal day care and extended maternity and paternity leave; they also recommend that all employment be part-time, so that men and women can share household and parenting responsibilities and women can seek fulfilling careers outside the home. The pamphlet sold so many copies that it was picked up and published the following year by Simon and Schuster—even though the authors had misgivings about trusting publication to a corporation and selling out to capitalism.

The twenty-first-century progressive left is, of course, a very different beast, with a very different set of priorities. It's safe to say that the struggle to end capitalism, in the US at least, is over. People struggle just to get medical care; the campaign to prevent medical experts taking control of their bodies is a luxury very few can afford. Women, and men, are more likely to be concerned about getting and keeping a job than with reducing their work hours. In this straitened, cautious atmosphere, we hear very little about maternity leave, let alone paternity leave. Women call for legislation to protect their "right" to pump breast milk in the workplace, and they are careful to balance that right against the needs of their employers. The left-wing critique of capitalism that loomed so large in the 1960s and 1970s is a relic, confined to a few die-hard academics and a small fringe of ageing hippies, the people who can be seen selling copies of the Communist newspaper outside university buildings. Even the Occupy movement has most often been described as a protest against corruption and inequality, but not capitalism.

Today, those on the progressive end of the political spectrum are more likely to think of themselves as having a social conscience rather than as class warriors. And that social conscience is less likely to be expressed through overtly political behavior like protests or boycotts than personal lifestyle choices such as eating locally sourced and organic food, buying fairtrade coffee, frequenting small independent bookstores, practicing yoga, cycling, recycling, driving hybrid vehicles, and, not least, breastfeeding.

Many of the lifestyle choices that define the hipster left today are primarily about consumption. These choices reflect a continuing commitment to the principle that "the personal is political," but they also seem to suggest that political power can be exercised through the market, with an eye to promoting more ethical consumption rather than fundamental change.

Which is not to say that many of these consumption choices don't bespeak a thoughtful critique of corporate practices. People who buy organic, hormone-free, and grass-fed meat, for example, are concerned about the effect of hormones and pesticides on their health. But they are also challenging the farming practices of the multibillion-dollar agribusiness corporations like Monsanto, Archer Daniels Midland, and DuPont, which produce enormous quantities of food through genetic modification, chemical fertilizers and pesticides, hormone injections, factory farming, and grain feeding. They operate on the assumption that eating is a political act because the large-scale, industrialized, corporate farming that grows and produces almost all of the food we eat jeopardizes not only our health but also the world around us, including the environment, the social fabric of rural America, and even the farming practices and survival of farmers as far away as Jamaica, Bangladesh, and Ghana.

Buying fair-trade coffee is another purchasing and consumption choice that sends a political message. The term *fair trade* is a critique of so-called free trade, which advances globalization on terms that have been widely recognized as significantly more beneficial to rich countries than to poor ones. The local food movement also expresses political commitments through personal consumption. Local food movements are prominent in every city in North America; they are advanced and sustained by magazines like *Edible*, local food websites and blogs, many restaurants, and the overwhelming popularity of farmers' markets.

Breastfeeding has also become part of this package of ethical consumption choices made by socially conscientious Americans. This has, of course, been true of breastfeeding since the Nestlé boycott in the 1970s. Breastfeeding advocacy linked activism around global poverty and infant mortality to struggles against corporate greed and unethical marketing practices. Even though the Nestlé boycott is about the dangers of formula in poor countries, the boycott is mostly carried out in developed countries and maintains our impression of breastfeeding as an alternative not only to formula but to big business in general.

Even more routinely, breastfeeding is acclaimed for its positive environmental impact. In fact *The Surgeon General's Call to Action to Support Breastfeeding*, published in 2010, identifies "environmental effects" as one important reason to choose breastfeeding. Human milk is a "renewable resource," and breastfeeding "reduces the carbon footprint by saving precious global resources and energy."

Mother Nature Network (www.mnn.com), a website dedicated to "the natural world, sustainable communities, and

simple food"—all under the heading of what it calls "responsible living"—includes a page on "green reasons why breastfeeding is the best feeding." Another organization dedicated to
green living, Care2, also explains why "breastfeeding is an environmental issue." Care2 focuses less on breast milk as a renewable food source and more on the waste produced by formula.
One organizer makes her point through some rough-and-ready
calculations, for example: "The 550 million cans of artificial
baby formula sold each year in the U.S. alone, stacked end to
end, would circle the earth one and a half times."

In fact, the connection between breastfeeding and the environment is repeated by almost all organizations dedicated to
environmentally friendly living. "After all," says one activist,
"you have to admit that when it comes to foods that are organic,
local, natural *and* free, *human breast milk* ticks all the boxes."
Breastfeeding advocacy groups are also quick to make the connection between breastfeeding and the environment, aware that
many women who breastfeed are also concerned about environmental degradation, waste, and greenhouse gas emissions.
As one self-identified environmentalist explained, "My decision
to breastfeed my babies was not just a personal decision but also
a planetary decision."

CHRISTIANS HAVE ALSO EMERGED AS forceful breastfeeding advocates. It turns out there are twenty-five references to breastfeeding in the Bible. Lamentations 4:3 says it is cruel not to
breastfeed: "Even the jackals draw out the breast, they give suck
to their young ones, but the daughter of my people has become
cruel, like the ostriches in the wilderness." In Joel 2:16, God
specifically mentions nursing mothers when he invites people
to a public congregation: "Gather the people, consecrate the

assembly; bring together the elders, gather the children, those nursing at the breast." A number of biblical references identify a child's age by whether or not he was weaned. In Thessalonians 2:7, the apostles liken their own dedication to God's followers to the devotion of a nursing mother toward her baby. The Bible also states explicitly that Naomi breastfed (Ruth 4:16), Moses was breastfed (Exodus 2:9), and Samuel was breastfed until he was old enough to go to temple (1 Samuel 1:23)—probably until he was four or five.

I wasn't familiar with these quotes because I'm a meticulous biblical scholar. I'm familiar with them now because I found them prominently featured on the many Christian breastfeeding websites. Conservative, fundamentalist, born-again, and evangelical Christians draw on biblical references like these to prove that God endorses breastfeeding and approves of nursing mothers. They advise mothers who are considering feeding their baby formula to turn to the Bible, which, they insist, makes an open and shut case for breastfeeding. In a quick twenty minutes on Google, I found twenty-three websites, mostly dedicated to Christian parenting, that drew directly on the Bible and listed every single biblical passage that mentioned breastfeeding to demonstrate that breastfeeding is not only God's will but part of "His divine plan."

Many Christian parenting websites also cite breastfeeding as evidence of intelligent design. Intelligent design is the creationist theory of the origin of the universe and the beginning of human life. It is a biblically inspired alternative to the big bang theory of the universe and to the theory of evolution. Many Christians believe that, as the Bible states in Genesis, God created the universe, and mankind, in his image. The basic idea of intelligent design is that the universe and all living things are too complex to be the result of a natural selection process. Instead, there must have been a designer, and that designer, they believe, was God.

In an article titled "Breastfeeding by Design," Heidi Bingham begins by stating, "Breastfeeding is God's design." Bingham identifies herself as a Christian, homeschooling, stay-at-home mom. Her website is dedicated to "Christian living." Bingham offers various pieces of evidence to support her claim, including "When Cain was born, God filled Eve's breasts with milk for him. He did not drop a case of formula in her pantry." A website called Gentle Christian Mothers echoes this sentiment. "We believe that Breastmilk is God's design in infant nutrition. Breastfeeding satisfies not only babies' hunger and thirst, but it also is a great way to pacify and comfort them."

Whereas these mothers are using the idea of intelligent design to support breastfeeding, the Institute for Creation Research, an organization whose goal is to "scientifically challenge the arguments used in support of evolution" and to "defend Genesis and refute evolution," invokes breastfeeding as proof of intelligent design. In a research paper called "Design in Infant Nutrition," Rex D. Russell, MD, argues that mother's milk is designed to change with the changing needs of her baby. A mother whose baby is born prematurely produces milk, he says, that has more of the nutrients a premature baby needs than that milk would have if the baby were full term. (This, by the way, is untrue.) He offers this evidence to refute the evolutionary logic of "survival of the fittest," which, he explains, would not support the survival of premature babies. He concludes, "Is there any way random chance (even controlled by "Mother Nature," "Mother Earth," or millions of mutations) could produce such an awesome product? If the mother's milk was not well-designed from the beginning, humankind would be extinct. Human milk cries the message of design! Thank the Creator!" It's an unusual conclusion for a scientific research paper.

Breastfeeding is also enlisted on behalf of another one of the Christian Right's signature issues—that families are made up of a man and a woman, each of whom has a distinct, biologically determined role to play in marriage. The point is straightforward. "When a man and woman marry, they take certain functional positions. Men are called to be the head of the household while women are to submit to them. The husband has the final authority, and responsibility, for what goes on in the home." Christian roles are firmly rooted in biology, which offers mothers two roles: to help her husband and bear children. Breastfeeding is proof that God opposes same-sex marriage, and it is also a way of carrying out God's will by adopting a specifically gendered role within a marriage. "God's plan for women is to be nurturers in the home and society. When we breastfeed we embrace our womanhood."

In the same way that many Christians believe that breastfeeding is integral to God's plan for how we are to live our lives, they also believe that the failure to breastfeed may be a violation or subversion of God's will. Feeding a baby formula is a sin. "If it's on your mind, ask yourself why you wish to bottle feed." If bottle feeding is on your mind, in fact, you may also be responsible for other digressions from Christian family values. "The rejection in our hearts of our womanly functions of pregnancy, childbirth and nursing is a root of homosexuality."

Part of the reason so many Christian organizations and websites have become so vocal about breastfeeding is that there has been some resistance to breastfeeding from the church, and from Christians, who are concerned with women's modesty and with the possibility that breastfeeding will provoke men to the sin of lust.

I mentioned earlier that Pope Francis recently weighed in on this debate—about whether Christian women should breast-feed as sanctioned in the Bible, or should avoid breastfeeding because it is immodest—on the side of breastfeeding. In January 2014, at a baptismal ceremony in the Sistine Chapel, the pope urged mothers to feed their babies if they cried "without thinking twice." He also told reporters he had encouraged another mother to feed her crying baby during a church service. Every major news service in the Western Hemisphere carried the news that the pope had endorsed breastfeeding in public and, specifically, in church.

No doubt the pope's support for breastfeeding will strengthen, and broaden, the perception that breastfeeding is a Christian issue. For some it is an expression of faith in God. God did it right the first time, and no amount of "tampering in a formula lab" will ever come close. Breastfeeding is also a way of living according to God's will and following Christ. If God provided mothers with milk to feed an infant, we should use it. One woman who identifies as a born-again Charismatic Evangelical explained her reason for breastfeeding in a manner that was uncannily similar to the way the environmentalist in the last section explained that breastfeeding was not only a personal decision but also a planetary decision: "For me, breastfeeding was not just a health-related choice, it was a God-inspired choice."

BREASTFEEDING, IT TURNS OUT, is never *just* breastfeeding. It's loaded with meaning for pretty much everyone who does it, not to mention those who don't. It sends a message about who we are and what we believe in. Still, the big surprise is not necessarily that breastfeeding has taken on so much meaning for many Americans but just *how many* different meanings it has and how many of these different meanings *directly contradict* one another.

Whereas feminists embrace breastfeeding as a symbol of empowerment, conservative Christians embrace it as a symbol of womanly submission. Other women breastfeed because it is a lifestyle choice that identifies them as people of conscience, concerned with issues like global warming, environmental degradation, unequal terms of trade between developing and developed nations, and growing inequality between the haves and have-nots. And finally there are those who breastfeed because it is a crucial component of their status as full-time mothers. Their dedication to parenting stands in as a symbol of the family's financial security and moral responsibility.

In short, these days breastfeeding offers common ground to many people who are unable to see eye to eye on just about any other issue. No wonder, then, that contemporary politicians have also embraced breastfeeding in large numbers. As a consensus issue, it has the potential to win them support from all sectors. By offering the moral high ground to almost everyone, breastfeeding has become a central and highly cherished component of contemporary American culture. Given its exalted status, it is perhaps not entirely surprising that many people remain powerfully committed to breastfeeding even once they begin to hear that its much-touted health benefits are considerably less impressive than we have been led to believe.

CHAPTER 3

Medical Research

L activism is a big tent that houses many different kinds of people. These people are so different that it's quite likely they disagree about almost every other issue, from abortion to climate change, Obamacare to gun control. And even though they all agree that breast is best, they do so for strikingly different reasons. For feminists it is an act of female empowerment; for Christians a symbol of womanly submission; for yuppies an affirmation of class status; and for hipsters a way to reduce the carbon footprint. It is also promoted—most often by policy makers and politicians—as a form of good citizenship, a way for women to save their country $13 billion a year in medical costs. These different perspectives reveal just how broad the consensus around breastfeeding has become.

And yet there can be little doubt that each of these constituencies have converged around breastfeeding for one reason in particular: they believe it will improve the health and well-being of their babies for years to come, possibly even forever. After all, that's not only what their physicians tell them, it's also what they hear from authoritative health-care organizations such as the American Academy of Pediatrics (AAP), the Centers for Disease Control and Prevention (CDC), and the World Health Organization (WHO). In the last two decades or so, the number of health advantages associated with breastfeeding has grown truly dazzling. Breastfeeding, or breast milk, is credited with reducing the risk of ear infections, gastrointestinal infections, lower respiratory tract infections, necrotizing enterocolitis, high blood pressure, obesity, cardiovascular disease, diabetes, asthma, allergies, cancer, celiac disease, Crohn's disease, eczema, infant mortality, and sudden infant death syndrome (SIDS). Breastfed babies are also said to have higher IQs and to be more emotionally secure.

That simple premise—that breastfeeding improves the health and well-being of both children and society—has shaped the lives of parents, breastfeeders and formula feeders alike, for decades. *But is that simple, powerful premise true? Does breastfeeding materially improve the health and well-being of babies and children?* After reading through a couple hundred medical journal articles on the impact of breastfeeding, I sought the expert opinion of Dr. Michael Kramer.

DR. KRAMER IS PROBABLY THE MOST prominent breastfeeding researcher in the world today. After receiving his medical degree from Yale University in 1978, he accepted a position in the Faculty of Medicine at McGill University, where he is now, almost forty years later, a professor in both the Department of Pediatrics and the Department of Epidemiology and Biostatistics. Kramer has published nearly four hundred articles in prestigious medical journals like the *Journal of the American Medical*

Association (JAMA), the *British Medical Journal (BMJ)*, *The Lancet, New England Journal of Medicine*, and *Pediatrics*, and he has received numerous coveted awards recognizing his professional accomplishments. The main reason I wanted to meet with him is that he is also the lead researcher on the Promotion of Breastfeeding Intervention Trial (PROBIT)—the largest and most authoritative study of the effects of breastfeeding to date.

Like many people who are giants in their fields, Kramer is unassuming, soft-spoken—and intense. His bearing is slightly rigid, as if he might have suffered a back injury, but Kramer speaks with impressive grace and candor. He recalls even the most obscure details of breastfeeding research without any apparent effort, and fluently translates complex medical research and statistics into ordinary language.

Kramer has a global reputation not only as a leading pediatrician but also as a breastfeeding advocate. He authored the very influential 2001 report that led WHO to change its infant-feeding recommendation from four to six months of exclusive breastfeeding to six months of exclusive breastfeeding. A review of the available evidence showed, he argued, that prolonged and exclusive breastfeeding had a positive impact on gastrointestinal infection and that breast milk was sufficient for a baby's nutritional needs up to six months of age. Kramer's wife breastfed their children, and his pride was evident when he told me his daughter-in-law was breastfeeding. On balance, he believes breastfeeding is a good thing.

But he doesn't believe breastfeeding is important enough to justify the zealotry of ardent lactivists. The PROBIT study has found no connection between breastfeeding and many of the benefits prominently attributed to it. In fact, even the benefits it *has* found have been fairly modest. At this point, Kramer still thinks breastfeeding makes a difference, but not one that is likely to be life defining.

By 2013, when I traveled to Montreal to meet with him, I was determined to get a more precise picture of the benefits of breastfeeding. Without ever really intending to, I had breastfed for a very long time. I did it partly because it was easy for me and partly because I couldn't figure out how to stop. But the main reason I breastfed for over fifty months is that it made me feel like I was doing at least one thing right. Now I really wanted to know: did all those hours count for anything?

The answer is *yes*—and *no*. Over the course of the last twenty years, breastfeeding has been credited with lowering the risks for an astonishing range of health outcomes, from ear infections to cancer. The list of reported benefits is so long that the Department of Health and Human Services (DHHS) published a recent document stating simply that: "Most experts agree the benefits of breastfeeding are endless." The truth, though, seems to be much closer to another recent statement by Dr. Annette Buyken, a doctor, nutritionist, and breastfeeding advocate. According to Buyken, there is "accumulating evidence that the overall effects of breastfeeding on later health outcomes are likely to be modest." The distance between the DHHS's claim that the benefits are "endless" and Buyken's concession that they are "modest" was confusing, to say the least. Many recent studies suggest that breastfeeding has no effect on many of the outcomes it has been associated with, like obesity and allergies, and that, even where it has an effect, as it does with infection, in a developed country with routine access to clean drinking water, that effect is not nearly as powerful as many of us have believed. Sigh.

ONE OF THE BIG PROBLEMS BREASTFEEDING researchers con-
front is that there is no easy way to gather reliable data. Kramer
is famous in part because he designed a study that brilliantly got
around this long-standing problem. For decades now, randomized controlled trials have been recognized as the gold standard of scientific research methods. But breastfeeding makes
trials difficult to engineer. As the name suggests, in a randomized controlled trial, people are randomly assigned to different
groups and each group receives a different treatment or protocol. Researchers then review the results to compare how each
group responds. In the case of breastfeeding, a randomized controlled study would involve dividing mothers into two groups,
one of which would be asked to breastfeed and the other to formula feed, and then checking to see if health outcomes among
babies from the two groups differ.

Randomized experiments, as we know them today, were
invented by a scientist and statistician named Ronald Fisher,
who devised a famous randomized trial called Lady Tasting
Tea. The lady in question, Muriel Bristol, was a botanist who
worked with Fisher at the Rothamsted Experimental Station in
Hertfordshire, England. Bristol claimed she could tell whether
milk or boiling water had been poured first into a cup of tea.
In the experiment, Ronald gave Muriel eight cups of tea—
four prepared with milk poured first, four with boiling water
poured first—and served them to her in random order. Fisher
calculated that the probability that she would guess all eight
cups correctly was one in seventy. But the greater the number
of cups Bristol identified correctly, the lower the chance that
she was just a lucky guesser. A colleague of Fisher's later reported that Bristol correctly identified all eight cups. The lady
knew her tea.

Randomized experiments designed to test the effect of something health related, like a medication or a diet, follow the same basic principle as the Lady Tasting Tea experiment. Most significantly, they randomly sort people into different groups to eliminate the possibility that a particular outcome could have been caused by a confounding factor—that is, a factor other than the particular medication or protocol that is being tested.

In the context of breastfeeding research, for example, smoking is a confounding factor. It turns out that mothers who breastfeed are also less likely to smoke. This means that if babies of mothers who breastfeed get fewer respiratory tract infections, it isn't possible to say with certainty whether that reduced rate of infection was due to the fact that their mothers breastfed or to the fact that they were nonsmokers. If, however, researchers were able to randomly assign mothers to breastfeeding or formula-feeding cohorts, they could ensure that potential confounding factors, like smoking, were also randomly distributed between the two groups. Only then would they be in a position to prove that breastfeeding, and not some other confounding factor, was responsible for a particular outcome.

But there has never been a randomized controlled trial of breastfeeding because the medical community has decided it would be unfeasible and unethical to perform one. It is unfeasible, presumably, because women have preferences about the way they feed their babies and would decline to participate in a study that would force them to cast these preferences aside. Forcing a woman to feed her child contrary to her preferences would also be unethical.

The conviction that randomized trials for breastfeeding are both unfeasible and unethical means that scientific research into the benefits of breastfeeding has been observational.

Observational studies compare outcomes between babies who were breastfed and babies who were formula fed without randomly assigning mothers and babies to those two different groups. The problem with this approach is that, especially in the US, mothers who breastfeed tend to have other things in common: for example, they are not only less likely to smoke but also less likely to work, more likely to have completed college, wealthier, and more likely to be married. Those similarities are all confounding factors; any one of them might be the real cause of health outcomes that might otherwise be attributed to breastfeeding.

In observational studies, scientists control for confounding factors by comparing outcomes among different subsets of the research cohort. If they are trying to control for smoking, they will compare breastfeeders who smoke with formula feeders who smoke, or nonsmokers with nonsmokers, so that the only difference between the two groups is what they feed their babies.

But the greater the number of factors that need to be controlled for, the harder it is to do that. To control for lots of potential confounding factors—smoking, education, and class, for example—you need to do a multivariate statistical analysis. Multivariate statistics is designed specifically to isolate and analyze more than one factor at a time, using sophisticated computer software. This type of multivariate analysis, though, can only be run using very large sample sizes. To deal with the problem of not having a large enough sample size, different studies control for different confounding factors—some control for income, some for education, and so on. And because they often measure those factors in different ways, they frequently reach different conclusions. That's one reason you end up with research that is "inconclusive" from a scientific perspective. Research outcomes contradict one another in part because different studies measure different things.

Observational studies are also problematic because they can only control for measurable things. But there may be some factors that are associated with breastfeeding, like "mothering style," that are almost impossible to measure, yet make a difference nonetheless. Finally, many observational studies, especially studies on long-term outcomes, rely on their subjects' memories. For example, adults who have diabetes or Crohn's disease might be asked whether they were breastfed and for how long. But memory is notoriously unreliable, and scientists automatically discount studies that rely on patient recall.

Kramer devised the PROBIT study back in 1992 and 1993 in an effort to move beyond the limitations of observational studies. At that point, there were well over twelve thousand citations for breastfeeding in the index of published medical research. But because all of these cited articles were vulnerable to the problems that plague observational research in general, the findings were not very coherent. Many studies did not even account for potential confounding factors. Studies that claimed to have discovered a benefit—such as a reduced risk of heart disease— were contradicted by other studies that found no benefit whatsoever. The science around breastfeeding was in desperate need of better research methods, and thanks to initial funding from the Canadian National Health Research and Development Program, UNICEF, the Thrasher Fund, and the European regional office of the World Health Organization, PROBIT was up and running by 1996. When I met with Kramer in his large corner office across the street from the Montreal Children's Hospital, on a bitterly cold day in December 2013, we talked about his famous study at length.

The PROBIT study hinges on Kramer's inspired strategy for getting around the problem of randomization in breast-feeding trials. Even if it was not feasible or ethical for research-ers to randomly assign individual women to breastfeeding or formula-feeding cohorts, Kramer hit on the idea that it *was* feasible to randomly assign *hospitals* to breastfeeding interven-tions. Hospitals that did not receive the intervention—in this case, breastfeeding promotion training—would follow their normal procedure, which meant that the trial would not make their patients any worse off than they would have been without it. Along with his collaborators from McGill and the University of Toronto, Kramer decided to conduct the study in Belarus, a small former Soviet Republic sandwiched between Poland and Russia.

Belarus was ideal for their purposes because although most new mothers initiated breastfeeding at birth, the vast majority introduced formula soon thereafter and had stopped breast-feeding entirely by three months. If the breastfeeding inter-vention worked, there should be a real difference in exclusivity and duration between the group of mothers who were subject to the intervention and those who were not. Belarus was also ideal because it was, in all important ways, a developed country, with high educational standards, a functional health-care sys-tem, and regular access to clean water. For all the reasons made clear through the Nestlé crisis, any study of the relative bene-fits of breast and formula feeding would have markedly differ-ent results in a developing country than it would in a developed country.

The PROBIT study recruited a remarkably large sample of more than seventeen thousand mother-infant pairs from thirty-one different hospitals that they randomly assigned to two different groups. In the sixteen hospitals and outpatient clinics that formed the experimental group, medical personnel were trained to help mothers in breastfeeding technique, encouraged the early initiation of breastfeeding, kept infants and mothers together after birth, and avoided supplementing breastfeeding with other liquids. The fifteen hospitals and clinics in the control group followed standard postpartum infant-care practices: supplementing breastfeeding with formula, enforcing a strict feeding schedule, and separating the baby from the mother after birth.

Although most mothers in both groups initiated breastfeeding, mothers in the experimental group were much more likely than mothers in the control group to still be breastfeeding at three, six, nine, and twelve months. At three months, for example, 45 percent of mothers who had delivered at hospitals that had received the intervention were still exclusively breastfeeding, compared with 7 percent of those who delivered at the other hospitals. PROBIT's first important finding was that training hospital staff to encourage new mothers to breastfeed was an effective way to achieve more exclusive and prolonged breastfeeding.

The medical community has identified PROBIT as the gold standard of breastfeeding research. Because of the way the trial was designed, the large number of subjects it includes, the fact that it follows a wide range of outcomes over time and has retained a large proportion of subjects in follow-up, PROBIT enjoys a high degree of credibility and visibility. In a *JAMA* assessment of the study, Dr. Ruth Lawrence, a pioneering pediatrician who founded the field of neonatology and specializes in neonatal nutrition at the University of Rochester Medical Center called Kramer's research "masterful" in both its design and execution. Lawrence has been a world-renowned expert on the benefits of breastfeeding since the 1950s, and she remains a force to be reckoned with even now in her eighties. When she calls a study masterful, people listen. Kramer had figured out how to work around the problem of randomization that had undermined the scientific validity of the entire enterprise of breastfeeding research up to that point. A lot of the most reliable and up-to-date information about the effect of breastfeeding on health outcomes comes from the PROBIT study.

As masterful as it is, however, PROBIT is only one study. A better picture of the state of breastfeeding research emerges from reading PROBIT alongside a few prominent and recent meta-analyses of breastfeeding research. A meta-analysis is a study that reviews and analyzes all of the published research on a particular topic—the relationship between breastfeeding and asthma, for example—to assess the findings of the research as a whole, rather than those of any individual study. Partly as a result of the methodological problems I've already described, many of these meta-analyses find the evidence indicating that breastfed babies have a lower risk of some particular illness or condition to be inconclusive or mixed. Although there are studies that find it does have certain benefits, others report no effect whatsoever. Only rarely does all of the evidence point in the same direction.

Meta-analyses are also useful because they evaluate the quality of the research that has been done on a particular topic in order to exclude poor quality studies. Poor quality studies may have included too few subjects for the statistical analysis to be genuinely meaningful. Statistical methods are only reliable if they are used on a sample that is large enough to accurately reflect the population it was drawn from. One study often cited to support the idea that breastfeeding reduces the risk of ADHD, for example, studied only fifty subjects. Some studies are of poor quality because they failed to control for potential confounding variables, or they controlled for the *wrong* confounding variables. I was surprised to learn that a large number of breastfeeding studies do not take confounding variables into account at all. Older studies also rarely distinguished between exclusive breastfeeding, mostly breastfeeding, and breastfeeding once a day. That lack of precision makes it hard to aggregate the data because each study is measuring a different breastfeeding practice. A number of meta-analyses have concluded that there is simply not enough good quality data to assess the effects of breastfeeding on some particular outcome.

Finally, scientific research in general is subject to a problem commonly known as publication bias. Studies that find no result, or no statistically relevant correlation between two variables (in this case between, say, breastfeeding and heart disease), are much less likely to be published, or even submitted for publication, than studies that do find a relationship. In October 2013, a cover article in *The Economist* reported a wide range of important flaws in medical research—the kind of flaws that seriously undermine the credibility of the research doctors use routinely to treat patients. According to the article, one of those flaws is that scientific journals prefer to publish positive results—even though negative results are much more likely to be accurate. In the last two decades, this particular publishing bias has become more common. Between 1990 and 2007, the proportion of published negative results dropped from 30 to 14 percent. Scientists have expressed concern that breastfeeding research is particularly vulnerable to publication bias.

So, keeping in mind the weaknesses and potential weaknesses of most of the research on breastfeeding, what does that research show?

THERE IS NO QUESTION THAT THE PROSPECT of wading through all the claims made on behalf of breastfeeding is daunting. And it's not just that the list is impossibly long. It's that everyone has a different list—and allegedly new benefits crop up almost every day. Where to begin? Everywhere we look, breast is best, for yet another reason.

I decided to start with the conspicuously *short* list of benefits touted by Latch On NYC, New York City's 2012 breastfeeding advocacy campaign: protection against diarrhea, pneumonia, and ear infections. The Latch On campaign was implemented under the direction of the health commissioner of the city of New York, Dr. Thomas Farley. Farley is a pediatrician who has spent most of his career working at the CDC and the Louisiana Office of Public Health. He spent months rebuilding the New Orleans health system after Hurricane Katrina.

Farley is also a powerful advocate of using public health initiatives to change people's behavior: "Now that science has beaten back infectious diseases like cholera, influenza, and polio, public health is largely reimagining itself to fight chronic diseases like obesity, hypertension, and high cholesterol." You do that, he believes, by making it harder for people to make bad choices. This is an idea that has gained a lot of traction lately, under the label Nudge Theory, which was popularized by Harvard law professor Cass Sunstein and Chicago economics professor Richard Thaler. Farley believes in using government policy to nudge people toward better health.

Farley is probably best known for his extremely controversial effort to ban New York City stores from selling supersize soft drinks. That initiative was struck down by the New York Supreme Court before it went into effect. But his ambitious breastfeeding initiative also garnered a great deal of attention, largely because of the coercive means it used to promote breastfeeding in hospitals. But compared to other breastfeeding advertising campaigns, New York City's ads were notably less grandiose in their account of the health benefits of breastfeeding.

After he stepped down as New York City Health Commissioner in 2013, Farley was appointed Tisch Distinguished Fellow in Public Health at Hunter College. Eight months later, we met to discuss the Latch On campaign at his Hunter College office, where he was writing a book on health policy under the Bloomberg administration. His office was on 63rd Street, just off Park Avenue, in a building that was once the home of Franklin and Eleanor Roosevelt. We met in FDR's old office, which still has his desk in it.

When I asked Dr. Farley why he had decided to focus on diarrhea, pneumonia, and ear infections, among all the possible health benefits on offer, he didn't beat around the bush. Those were the areas where the research seemed most solid. As a pediatrician, he didn't feel comfortable making any broader claims for the benefits of breastfeeding.

Even here, however, the evidence is mixed. The initial results of the PROBIT study, published in *JAMA* in 2001, confirmed that breastfeeding reduced the incidence of gastrointestinal infection, in this case from 13 to 9 percent. By following up with babies breastfed for three or six months, PROBIT also concluded that the protective effects of breastfeeding exist only while a mother is actually breastfeeding and for about two weeks after she stops. On the other hand, the PROBIT study found that breastfeeding had no effect on ear infections or respiratory tract infections.

Kramer himself doubts the veracity of those negative results, however. He believes breastfeeding *does* in fact affect the risk of infection. Scientists, he says, have figured out exactly how the molecules in breast milk protect against infection. "We can see in vitro and in animal models how they work. Those mechanisms are pretty well worked out." Milk oligosaccharides and lactoferrin, both of which are present in breast milk, protect against bacterial and viral infections.

There are two reasons that PROBIT may have found that babies in the intervention group had no fewer cases of ear and respiratory infections than babies from the control group. First, most babies in both groups were actually breastfed for some period of time. Second, women in Belarus have long maternity leaves, and most babies in Belarus simply do not get ear or respiratory infections because they do not go to day care. That second explanation also accounts for the fact that only 13 percent of babies in Belarus suffered any gastrointestinal infections at all. In the United States, that number is closer to 60 percent.

If, however, breastfeeding protects against ear and respiratory tract infections in the US, what is the extent of its protective effect? Dr. David Meyers, the director of the US government's Agency for Healthcare Research and Quality (AHRQ), answered that question in a speech that was later printed in the medical journal *Breastfeeding Medicine*. Ruth Lawrence, the editor of the journal, explained in a footnote that Meyers's speech would help "put science into perspective in everyday life."

Meyers intended his speech to drive home how critical breast-feeding is to children's health. But when Meyers addressed the issue of ear and respiratory tract infections head on, the results were far less impressive than I had expected.

According to Meyers, "the evidence suggests that for every six children who are exclusively breastfed for six months of life, one of them will not have an ear infection that he or she would otherwise have had." The numbers for respiratory tract infections—like pneumonia—were even more underwhelming. "At least 26 infants will have to breastfeed exclusively for four or more months to prevent one infant from hospitalization."

Six women have to spend six months exclusively breastfeeding to prevent one ear infection? And that benefit is more than likely going to affect *someone else's* baby?! Conservatively speaking, that's about 5,400 hours of breastfeeding to prevent one ear infection; 15,600 hours of breastfeeding to prevent a case of pneumonia. I can't help thinking that Dr. Meyers must be doing a different cost-benefit analysis than most mothers would do. Of course ear infections are no fun. They make babies cranky and miserable, and nobody gets much sleep. But they're not life threatening either. It is at least arguable that preventing *one* ear infection isn't important enough to justify 5,400 hours of breastfeeding.

Breast milk may also reduce the risk of another type of infection: necrotizing enterocolitis (NEC), a potentially deadly intestinal infection. This is a rare condition that affects only one in four thousand babies, almost always preterm infants. The AHRQ meta-analysis concluded that there is a "marginally statistically significant association between breast milk feeding and a reduction in the risk of NEC." Based on that assessment, many neonatal units have adopted a combination of late-onset, slow, and continuous drip feeding with human milk as a standard protocol for feeding very premature babies.

On balance, breastfeeding does seem to make a modest difference in the risk of infection. The evidence of a link between breastfeeding and eczema, asthma, allergies, SIDS, type 2 diabetes, leukemia, cardiovascular disease, Crohn's disease, celiac disease, behavioral disorders, and intelligence is, however, mixed or inconclusive.

The initial PROBIT study corroborated a link between breastfeeding and atopic eczema among infants, reducing the incidence from 6.3 to 3.3 percent. A PROBIT follow-up study, conducted when the children were six and a half years old, showed no difference between the two groups. The PROBIT study also found that breastfeeding had no effect on asthma or allergies. In fact, babies who were breastfed were slightly *more* likely to have allergic symptoms than those who were formula fed.

Unfortunately, evidence of a connection between breastfeeding and SIDS, which is undoubtedly the most important outcome to be associated with breastfeeding, is also fairly contradictory. I lay out the evidence at some length here because it is so important, and so that the reader can draw her own conclusions.

Although the incidence of SIDS dropped dramatically following the 1992 AAP recommendation and campaign to have children sleep on their backs, there are still 2,300 cases of SIDS every year in the United States. Doctors believe that SIDS is caused by a combination of factors: some babies are born with a defect in the part of the brain that controls arousal and breathing; babies born premature are at increased risk of SIDS because that part of their brain is immature; and environmental stress can interfere with a baby's breathing or oxygen levels. Everyone agrees that the most important recommendations for reducing the risk of SIDS are putting the baby to sleep on his or her back, putting the baby to sleep in a crib, avoiding the use of pillows, blankets, or bumpers that could impede the flow of oxygen, and avoiding smoking during pregnancy. If these risks were eliminated, SIDS experts calculate that the incidence of SIDS could drop from 1 in 2,000 babies to 1 in 10,000 babies—fewer than four hundred deaths per year in the United States.

Whether breastfeeding could reduce that number even further is a matter of contention. Doctors who specialize in SIDS have long claimed it would not. In 2005, the AAP convened the Task Force on Sudden Infant Death Syndrome and published recommendations for the prevention of SIDS. Those recommendations focused almost exclusively on the risk factors identified above.

At that point, the task force reported that "factors associated with breastfeeding, but not breastfeeding" were related to SIDS and concluded that "although breastfeeding is beneficial and should be promoted for many reasons, the task force believes that the evidence is insufficient to recommend breastfeeding as a strategy to reduce SIDS." Another task force reaffirmed that conclusion in 2009.

In 2011, however, a new task force on SIDS included breastfeeding among its recommendations for reducing the risk of SIDS. The following year, a task force in Australia reviewed the literature on breastfeeding and SIDS and found that the evidence of a link was "inconsistent." That task force decided *against* including breastfeeding among its recommendations for reducing SIDS. A subsequent meta-analysis concluded, on the other hand, that research *does* show an association between breastfeeding and SIDS, and the AHRQ meta-analysis also found an association.

And yet researchers have not yet figured out *how* breastfeeding could lower the risk of SIDS. Breastfeeding seems very unlikely to have an impact on any underlying defect in the brain that weakens the arousal reflex, or on the maturity of that part of the brain. Nor will it prevent any obstruction in the flow of oxygen to the baby. On the other hand, research shows that roughly half of SIDS victims had symptoms of a slight infection in the days before death. In some, though clearly not all cases, SIDS may be associated with infection, or with an unusual host response to infection, although scientists have yet to find an association between SIDS and any particular bacteria or virus. If there is a link between breastfeeding and SIDS, it may be because breastfeeding reduces the risk of respiratory infection. But when I asked Dr. Farley why he hadn't included reducing the risk of SIDS among the Latch On campaign claims for the benefits of breastfeeding, he raised one eyebrow. "Yes, we did consider SIDS," he admitted, "But there, too, I thought the science was pretty shaky." It seems as if the AAP might concur. The organization's website summarizes the AAP policy statement on breastfeeding and human milk by listing ten benefits for which it claims there is evidence of a link to breastfeeding. The list does not include SIDS.

Whether breastfeeding has an effect on type 2 diabetes—the type of diabetes that is associated with obesity and inactivity—is also complicated. In 2006, the *American Journal of Clinical Nutrition* published a meta-analysis of the research on the effect of breastfeeding on type 2 diabetes. The authors excluded seventeen of the twenty-four studies they found on breastfeeding and type 2 diabetes because they were of poor quality. Six of the remaining seven studies found that breastfeeding was associated with a reduced risk of type 2 diabetes.

But only three of those studies controlled for confounding variables that are known to be strongly associated with type 2 diabetes: maternal weight, socioeconomic status, and infant weight at birth. Two of those three studies were conducted among Native Americans, who are at greater risk of type 2 diabetes than the rest of the population and may not be a representative sample. Most crucially, none of the studies controlled for maternal diabetes, which is quite a glaring omission. The authors of the meta-analysis concluded that more studies would be necessary to determine whether there really is an independent breastfeeding effect on type 2 diabetes. If there is, they estimate that 5 percent of diabetes cases could be attributed to lack of breastfeeding, which, they point out, "is modest compared with the potential benefits of reductions in obesity in later life."

The evidence for an association between breastfeeding and a reduced risk of acute lymphoblastic leukemia (ALL) is also equivocal. ALL is a specific type of childhood leukemia that strikes roughly 2,800 people under the age of twenty in the United States every year. This means that the risk of contracting this type of leukemia is less than one in twenty-five thousand; but roughly 280 children die of this disease every year.

Out of a total of ten "quality-rated" studies of breastfeeding and ALL, six were eliminated from meta-analysis because of poor quality. Of the remaining four, two were rated "fair" and two, "good." One good and one fair study found that breastfeeding had a protective effect, and the other good and fair studies found no association. The overall conclusion of the AHRQ meta-analysis was that "there are few high-quality studies to inform an important question for parents as to whether it is possible to reduce the risk of childhood leukemia by breast-feeding, and those few studies disagree." At this point, they just don't know if breastfeeding makes a difference.

There is only one study that has identified links between breastfeeding and Hodgkin's disease, and breastfeeding and neuroblastoma. The authors of that study cautioned that the correlation they found was very small and may not be causal.

Although some studies have also suggested that breastfeeding decreases the risk for cardiovascular disease, the author of one meta-analysis concluded that "the literature is mixed." Another meta-analysis reported that most studies of the association between breastfeeding and Crohn's disease have either "failed to achieve statistically significant results or found no association at all." It's unlikely that breastfeeding protects against celiac disease. And although a small Israeli study found that breastfeeding was protective against ADHD, the PROBIT study found that breastfeeding had no effect on childhood behavior, including hyperactivity and behavioral problems.

On the other hand, the PROBIT study did find that breast-feeding had an effect on cognitive development. I was delighted. Even if breastfeeding wouldn't have much effect on my children's health, I was glad to find it would make them smarter.

Ultimately, however, Kramer cautioned me not to get too carried away. Although PROBIT found that, at age six and a half, breastfed children scored seven points higher for verbal IQ, three points higher for performance IQ, and six points higher for full-scale IQ, Kramer nonetheless described these effects as "modest." Basically, he said "we shouldn't expect that you're going to be producing Mozarts or Einsteins just because you're breastfeeding." During the course of our conversation, he further qualified the results by explaining that "the verbal IQ results were not very precise because the confidence interval was quite wide."

In statistics, a confidence interval basically tells you how likely it is that the results you got were accurate. In this case, the results were weaker than they appeared to be because the IQ tests were conducted by different pediatricians at different sites, and different pediatricians produced systematically different results. Some pediatricians consistently assessed all their patients higher, or lower, than an average would predict, and those tendencies produced systematically different results by clinic, not only by individual child. Those systematic variations reduced the "power" of the study because the researchers essentially had to control for the pediatricians. Given all this, Kramer's own interpretation of PROBIT's IQ result was tempered. "Although it was statistically significant, if you asked me if I thought the real effect was that big, I would say probably not. It's too big an effect."

Kramer's team is currently conducting follow-up tests to improve the objectivity of their measures of cognitive intelligence by using computers, rather than pediatricians, to collect data on the children at age sixteen. "It'll be a little embarrassing if we find nothing. Then we won't know if we didn't measure it right the first time, or if the effect has just faded over time. Either way it will be disappointing," said Kramer. Since those results won't be out until the end of 2015, the jury is still out on whether my many hundreds of hours of breastfeeding will boost my children's test scores.

The rest of the literature on breastfeeding and cognitive development could reasonably be described as all over the map. There is disagreement over whether breastfeeding has an effect on intelligence, disagreement over how considerable that effect is, and disagreement over the real cause of the potential effect. A recent Brazilian study that garnered a lot of attention in the US found that breastfeeding not only improved IQ but also led to higher income later in life. But two prominent studies that have managed to eliminate confounding factors by comparing siblings (one breastfed, one formula-fed) within the same household, published respectively in 2006 and 2014, both found that breastfeeding had no effect on academic achievement or intelligence. The AHRQ meta-analysis concluded point-blank that "there was no relationship between breastfeeding in term infants and cognitive performance." So, believe what you want about breastfeeding and intelligence; there's evidence to support you either way. Those three or four IQ points probably aren't worth going to the mat over.

In other cases the evidence is no longer mixed: it decisively disproves a breastfeeding benefit. Recent research and reviews have confirmed that there is no connection between breastfeeding and blood pressure, and the PROBIT study found that breastfeeding had no effect on dental health.

Breastfeeding also appears to have no impact on type 1 diabetes. PROBIT did not study this outcome, but the AHRQ meta-analysis did. Their review of the research found that studies that relied on a patient's memory identified a correlation between breastfeeding and a reduced risk of type 1 diabetes. But studies that used infant-feeding records, rather than memory, found no association between type 1 diabetes and breastfeeding. A 2003 study published in *JAMA* supports this finding.

The AHRQ meta-analysis also reviewed research on the effect of breastfeeding on cancer, concluding that there is "little evidence that breastfeeding was associated with acute non-lymphomoblastic leukemia, non-Hodgkins lymphoma, central

nervous system cancers, malignant germ cell tumors, juvenile
bone tumors, or other solid cancers." At this point, the possibility of an association between breastfeeding and these cancers
has essentially been dismissed by the AHRQ.

Even the much-touted impact of breastfeeding on obesity
had been pretty roundly debunked, even *before* it was widely
publicized. In the last few years, the idea that breastfeeding
protects against obesity has gone viral—especially after Michelle Obama embraced breastfeeding as part of her Let's Move
campaign in 2011. But the fact remains that a number of different studies, published in top-ranking medical journals in
2003, 2005, 2007, 2011, 2012, 2013, and 2014, have shown decisively that breastfeeding has no protective effect against obesity.
Kramer believes this is what scientists would call a robust finding. He says he would be *very* surprised if it was disproven by
future studies. With respect to obesity, the *BMJ* has concluded
"we will have to look elsewhere for an answer to childhood
obesity." Almost all studies of breastfeeding and weight have
reached the same conclusion—that the strongest predictor of
the weight of the child is the weight of the mother.

SO WHAT, ULTIMATELY, is a parent to make of all these different
claims and counterclaims? What exactly does breastfeeding offer in the way of health and cognitive benefits?

On balance it seems that breastfeeding does appear to offer
modest protection against four types of infection: ear, gastrointestinal, and respiratory infections and necrotizing enterocolitis. The evidence that breastfeeding protects against eczema,
asthma, allergies, SIDS, type 2 diabetes, leukemia, cardiovascular disease, Crohn's disease, celiac disease, behavioral disorders,
and that it increases intelligence, is inconclusive or mixed. And,

there is strong evidence that breastfeeding has *no* effect on obesity, blood pressure, most cancers, ADHD and other behavioral disorders, type 1 diabetes, or dental health.

If you've spent months and months breastfeeding, as I have, this long list of findings is pretty disappointing. Maybe you breastfed because you loved it, or because you got that endorphin high some women describe. But still, at some level you were most likely breastfeeding because you believed what you were told: that it would bring "significant" benefits to your children.

Maybe the problem lies in part with the difference in the way the term *significant* is used in statistical analysis and the way it is used in common language. In statistics, "significant" does not mean big or important; it means something more like *noticeable* or *likely to be real and not an artificial result of statistical manipulation.* In medical research, a "significant effect" might still be a very small effect. But when we laypeople hear that something has a "significant effect" we tend to assume that the effect is large and important. And if that is what we thought, we are likely to be very disappointed. Breastfeeding is simply not the panacea new parents hope to find to protect their precious and vulnerable baby.

The question is why, then, so many of the country's leading health organizations and policy makers continue to behave as if it is.

CHAPTER 4

The End of Choice

Maya was riding the subway to her son's day care one morning in the fall of 2012. As they crossed the Manhattan Bridge into Brooklyn, she pointed out a tugboat on the river below and started feeding her son a bottle of breast milk she had expressed that morning, just before leaving the house. She knew it wouldn't be snack time at his day care for another couple of hours, and she didn't want him to get hungry. Focused on her baby and thinking also about the workday ahead, Maya hadn't noticed that she was sitting directly under a poster advertising the benefits of breast milk. It was only when she looked up to check which subway stop they were approaching that she noticed several passengers sending her unmistakably dirty looks. Was her stroller taking up too much room? She pulled it in a little closer to her seat. As a man got off at the DeKalb Avenue station, he turned back to yell at her, "Can't you read?" Maya was still staring at the closing door, completely bewildered, when a woman across the aisle shook her head disapprovingly and said, almost under her breath: "People like you shouldn't have kids."

The posters that plastered New York City subways and bus shelters with messages about the health benefits of breast milk were part of Latch On NYC, the city-wide initiative to promote breastfeeding launched by Mayor Michael Bloomberg in 2012 and spearheaded by Dr. Farley, the New York City Health Commissioner under Mayor Bloomberg. The posters featured a picture of a white, black, or Hispanic baby along with three different claims about the health benefits of breastfeeding: "Breast milk lowers baby's risk of diarrhea." "Breast milk lowers baby's risk of ear infections." "Breast milk lowers baby's risk of pneumonia." The posters were only one element of Bloomberg's Latch On NYC campaign—and, as we'll see, far from its most controversial one. But isolated experiences such as Maya's offer a glimpse of the zealotry and social shaming that breastfeeding sometimes elicits—and, sometimes, even encourages. Some of the passengers on the subway that day may even have felt obliged, as citizens, to speak out, believing, as the New York City Department of Health's message implied, that this bottle-wielding mother was not only endangering her child's health but imposing public health costs on "all of us." Nobody stopped to ask her what was in the bottle.

IN THE HISTORY OF BREASTFEEDING advocacy in this country, the year 2012 looms large. That was when the American Academy of Pediatrics (AAP) released an official statement identifying breastfeeding as a "public health issue and not only a lifestyle." Media outlets including *Time*, the *Huffington Post*, and the *New York Times* responded immediately. The AAP's declaration was big news. By identifying breastfeeding as a public health issue, the AAP had decided that infant feeding was a matter of public interest. Danielle Rigg, the cofounder of the breastfeeding advocacy organization Best for Babes, summarized the implications of the AAP's decision: "In framing it that way, [breastfeeding] becomes all of our responsibility—not just moms."

By making breastfeeding "all of our responsibility," the AAP's statement effectively transformed breastfeeding from a personal parental choice into a civic obligation—one we are all responsible for ensuring that moms fulfill. Interviewed by *Time* magazine about the policy statement, its coauthor, Dr. Richard Schanler, made this obligation explicit: "It's not should I or shouldn't I. Of course you should." When I spoke to him on the phone in August 2014, he made the same point: "This is a health issue for the better health of our infants, so why are we just leaving it up to the whim of the family to do whatever they feel like? This is not a lifestyle choice, it's something that's important that we advocate for our children."

By 2012, the decision to identify breastfeeding as a public health issue had in fact been in the works for a long time. In 1984, then surgeon general C. Everett Koop initiated the public dialogue about breastfeeding in the United States by convening a Surgeon General's Workshop on Breastfeeding and Human Lactation. That workshop was held at the University of Rochester and chaired by Dr. Ruth Lawrence—whom we encountered earlier as the highly respected breastfeeding specialist and advocate who identified Dr. Kramer's PROBIT study as "masterful." Koop's workshop attempted to align US government policy with international opinion inasmuch as it identified breastfeeding promotion as a national priority. But it was still fairly subdued. The overall tone was set in the report's conspicuously tentative first line: "Breastfeeding is believed to provide substantive advantages to both the mother and the infant."

The AAP published its first policy statement on breastfeeding in 1997. The Department of Health and Human Services (DHHS) followed suit shortly thereafter, publishing its first *HHS Blueprint for Action on Breastfeeding* in 2000. The blueprint urged doctors, employers, and child-care facilities to formulate policies that would encourage women to breastfeed longer. In 2010, then surgeon general Dr. Regina Benjamin issued *The Surgeon General's Call to Action to Support Breastfeeding*. Benjamin's call to action stated that the 2000 blueprint had "declared breastfeeding to be a key public health issue in the United States." In so doing, Benjamin managed simultaneously to attribute to the blueprint a claim that it hadn't made—namely, that breastfeeding is a public health issue—while, paradoxically, also lamenting that "for too long, breastfeeding has received insufficient national attention as a public health issue."

The 2010 call to action was nonetheless explicit about why it considered breastfeeding to be a public health issue and not simply a matter of personal and individual choice. Like most breastfeeding initiatives, the surgeon general's call begins by describing the health, psychological, and economic benefits breastfeeding offers individual infants, mothers, and families. She then goes on to use those benefits to explain the high cost that *not* breastfeeding imposes on society as a whole.

As with any clear-eyed cost-benefit analysis, breastfeeding is recommended here as an efficient practice that saves the government and its citizens money. "Better infant health means fewer health insurance claims, less employee time off to care for sick children, and higher productivity, all of which concern employers." The report goes on to cite a 2001 study that alleged that breastfeeding would save American taxpayers $3.6 billion annually. The surgeon general explained that this number includes the costs borne by families themselves, such as formula; the costs borne by insurance companies and therefore passed along to everyone else; the costs borne by employers, such as sick days taken by parents caring for sick children; and the costs borne by society as a whole through the loss of productivity associated with premature death caused, apparently, by formula feeding.

In an essay titled "Making the Case: Effective Language for Breastfeeding Advocacy," Dr. Melissa Bartick explains that identifying breastfeeding as a public health issue is an effective way to defuse the argument that parents should have a right to choose how to feed their babies. Bartick is a prolific and ardent lactivist and the director of the Massachusetts Breastfeeding Coalition, a nonprofit advocacy group that hosts an annual conference, publishes and disseminates a breastfeeding resource guide, and coordinates the work of breastfeeding advocates across Massachusetts. Breastfeeding, Bartick explains, "is a public health issue, just like smoking, safe sex, and seatbelts. This message removes the baggage of your audience's personal breastfeeding issues, and is an effective antidote to the language of 'choice' so popular with our opponents." She advises lactivists to counter the choice argument with claims about "marketing" and "profits" and to "avoid the word choice altogether."

Bartick also instructs advocates to "cite the risks of not breast-feeding, both to mothers and to children, both for acute and chronic illnesses" and to "include specific statistics rather than just general language about risk." As the essay continues, "saying babies who are formula-fed have double the risk of diarrhea sounds informative and scientific." She's right. It does. But double is only a significant number if those babies live in rural Afghanistan. The PROBIT study found that breastfeeding reduced the incidence of gastrointestinal infections from 13 percent to 9 percent. Not only is 13 percent not "double" 9 percent, but the numbers are so small that even saying it reduces the risk by one-third overstates the effect of breastfeeding on diarrhea.

In 2011, Bartick took an important step in her crusade to position breastfeeding as a public health issue. She and an IT consultant named Arnold Reinhold published an article in the medical journal *Pediatrics* claiming that the failure to breast-feed generated an annual cost of $13 billion and caused 911 deaths. This article revised the 2001 report cited by the surgeon general by expanding the list of illnesses that would be avoided by breastfeeding, increasing the percentage of women who should be breastfeeding, and updating the cost to 2011 dollars. As Bartick and her coauthor claimed: "If 90% of US families could comply with medical recommendations to breastfeed exclusively for 6 months, the United States would save $13 billion per year and prevent an excess 911 deaths, nearly all of which would be in infants."

Bartick's method for arriving at this figure merits careful attention. First, she assumes that breastfeeding lowers the risk of ten different conditions or diseases: necrotizing enterocolitis, ear infections, gastroenteritis, lower respiratory tract infections, atopic dermatitis, SIDS, childhood asthma, childhood leukemia, type 1 diabetes, and childhood obesity. But as we saw in the previous chapter, the evidence of a link between breastfeeding and many of these health outcomes is mixed or inconclusive. There is strong evidence that breastfeeding has *no* preventive effect on asthma, obesity, or type 1 diabetes. The evidence of a link between breastfeeding and SIDS, leukemia, and atopic dermatitis is mixed. Even the surgeon general's 2010 report acknowledged that "almost all the data (regarding the health benefits of breastfeeding) were gathered from observational studies. Therefore the associations described in the report do not necessarily represent causality." Bartick's study, on the other hand, assumes that those associations *do* imply causality.

But Bartick didn't stop there. To make the additional case that exclusive breastfeeding for six months would avert 911 deaths per year, Bartick made the assumption that the children who died of these diseases and illnesses would have lived, if only they had been breastfed. Yet the fact is that breastfeeding probably has little or no effect on most of these health outcomes. Even if it did, there is absolutely *no* medical evidence to suggest that—in a developed country with regular access to clean drinking water—breastfeeding makes the difference between life and death. Except possibly in the case of necrotizing enterocolitis, breastfeeding in the US does not have the life-saving potential it can have in the developing world.

Finally, Bartick reached the astonishing sum of $13 billion by estimating the hypothetical dollar costs of the illnesses and deaths that could have been prevented by breastfeeding—and then adding on the projected lost lifetime earnings of the 911 dead babies. Notwithstanding the questionable evidence and various leaps of logic embedded in their calculations, Bartick and Reinhold's study was picked up and enthusiastically reported by seventeen major news organizations, all of which accepted their claims at face value.

By the time the AAP issued its policy statement in 2012, it really wasn't marking out new territory. It was, to extend the metaphor, planting its own flag in territory that had long since been explored. Still, its flag mattered. The AAP is, after all, the professional association of pediatricians and the most authoritative voice the US has when it comes to our children's health. The policy statement was published in *Pediatrics*, the AAP's medical journal. Its coauthors, Dr. Arthur Eidelman, a pediatrician and professor of pediatrics at Hebrew University in Jerusalem, and Dr. Richard Schanler, a neonatologist at Long Island Jewish Medical Center and North Shore University Hospital, are both respected figures in their field.

But Eidelman and Schanler's statement declaring breastfeeding a public health issue was at odds with a great deal of contemporary research. Their statement asserted that breastfeeding reduces the risk of almost all of the health outcomes that have ever been associated with it: not only ear infections, pneumonia, and diarrhea, but also allergies, celiac disease, inflammatory bowel disease, SIDS, dermatitis, types 1 and 2 diabetes, leukemia, necrotizing enterocolitis, lymphoma, and obesity. The report also includes a table that specifies the exact percentages by which breastfeeding reduces the risk of each outcome. Exclusive breastfeeding, it says, reduces the risk of ear infections by 50 percent. It reduces the risk of obesity by 24 percent. Celiac disease? 52 percent.

I spoke to Schanler by phone about the policy statement in August 2014. I was surprised by its timing. Why was the AAP identifying breastfeeding as a public health issue just as evidence was accumulating that the health benefits of breastfeeding were probably modest? How did Schanler and Eidelman decide which sources to trust in making their various claims? Schanler directed the question back to me. "Well, how do *you* choose your sources? I just drew on the best research. For policy statements you try to look at meta-analyses and not single, small studies. Try to pick large well-respected studies."

But as I read the policy statement, I noticed that Schanler and his coauthor did not just pick "large well-respected studies" and rely on them consistently. In fact, they drew on numerous studies in a fairly selective manner. The official AAP policy statement drew heavily on the highly regarded Agency for Healthcare Research and Quality (AHRQ) meta-analysis I referred to in Chapter 3, identifying it as a source for almost all of the policy statement's claims. In many cases, however, the AHRQ meta-analysis was much less positive than the AAP policy statement. In those cases, Schanler and his coauthor supplemented it with a wide range of sources—often single, small studies that reported strikingly positive results.

For example, the AHRQ meta-analysis identified the research on asthma and leukemia as "equivocal." Drawing on other research, the AAP statement reported that breastfeeding reduced the risk of leukemia by 20 percent, and of asthma by 26 to 40 percent.

The AHRQ meta-analysis also concluded that most research on breastfeeding and types 1 and 2 diabetes "should be interpreted with caution" because it had not adequately adjusted for confounders that are known to be associated with diabetes. In fact, as I mentioned in the previous chapter, the AHRQ meta-analysis found that studies that relied on infant-feeding records, rather than memory, found no association between type 1 diabetes and breastfeeding. Drawing on other research, the AAP policy statement reported straightforwardly that breastfeeding reduced the risk of type 1 diabetes by 30 percent and type 2 diabetes by 40 percent.

Similarly, the AHRQ meta-analysis stated that "there was no relationship between breastfeeding in term infants and cognitive performance." Turning next to the PROBIT study, the AAP policy statement reported that "outcomes of intelligence scores and teacher's ratings are significantly greater in breastfed infants." But the statement did not mention any of the other

PROBIT findings, many of which were negative. It made no mention of the PROBIT findings on obesity, for example. The policy statement instead simply asserts that breastfeeding reduces the risk of obesity by 24 percent.

The AAP's 2012 declaration that breastfeeding is a public health issue not only received lots of media attention; it remains a highly influential document for pediatricians. It serves as the basis for numerous AAP publications about breastfeeding management and infant nutrition, including the AAP *Breastfeeding Handbook for Physicians*, the AAP Breastfeeding Residency Curriculum, and basically every other AAP publication regarding breastfeeding and human milk. The AAP policy statement is where pediatricians and other infant-care specialists go to learn best practices and to get a snapshot of current research. The report states clearly that it is the responsibility of pediatricians to advocate and support breastfeeding.

IN THE SAME YEAR THAT *Pediatrics* published the AAP policy statement, New York City launched one of the most far-reaching, and ultimately controversial, breastfeeding advocacy campaigns ever contemplated in the United States. The Latch On NYC campaign was in keeping with a number of other high-profile public health initiatives implemented by the activist Bloomberg administration. In 2003, Bloomberg extended New York's public smoking ban to all buildings, including bars and nightclubs. In 2006, New York City banned restaurants and food vendors from using trans fats. In 2012, Bloomberg announced his plan to ban supersized sodas, limiting the size of sodas to sixteen ounces. Every single one of these initiatives was controversial. In fact, the supersized soda ban was ultimately struck down by the New York Supreme Court before it went into effect, on the grounds that the city had exceeded the scope of its regulatory authority.

Latch On NYC was also controversial, not least because it was widely perceived to infringe on a mother's right to choose how to feed her baby. The program required hospitals to restrict access to formula by keeping it under lock and key, as they do in the case of prescription drugs. It also prohibited breastfeeding mothers from using formula as a supplement unless it was medically indicated and documented on the infant's medical chart. The specific protocol instructed nurses to: "Assess if breastfeeding is going well and encourage the mother to keep trying. Provide education and support to mothers who are experiencing difficulties. If the mother still insists on receiving formula, document it in the chart along with the reason and distribute only the amount of formula needed for the feeding."

Latch On NYC also includes sixty-four specific instructions for interactions between medical personnel and new mothers in hospitals, mostly geared toward making it very hard for a mother to feed her baby formula. One enthusiastic administrator at Staten Island University Hospital made this logic explicit: "The key to getting more moms to breast-feed is making the formula less accessible. This way, the RN has to sign out the formula like any other medication. The nurse's aide can't just go grab another bottle."

A blogger on the popular feminist website Feministe redescribed this strategy in her own words, "So a mother asks for a bottle, and the recommended response is to first encourage her to breastfeed, then educate her on why breastfeeding is a better choice, and then if she 'still insists' distribute enough formula for one feeding. And then repeat that every time the infant needs another bottle. That's not supporting the choice to breastfeed, that's shaming mothers for bottlefeeding."

Beyond the restrictions imposed on new mothers in hospitals, the Latch On NYC initiative included the poster advertising campaign I mentioned earlier. Along with information about the effect of breast milk on pneumonia, ear infections, and diarrhea, every poster included the following slogan: "It's your right to feed your baby only breast milk and get the support you need." That strange sentence bears repeating: *It's your right to feed your baby only breast milk and get the support you need.*

The distorted logic of the slogan says a lot. What it does not say explicitly, but clearly implies, is that it is *not* "your" right to feed your baby anything other than, or in addition to, breast milk. It also logically implies that parents who have adopted a baby, or gay dads, or a woman who cannot produce breast milk have a right to demand breast milk for their babies. That sort of inclusiveness would be very encouraging, but I doubt that's the message the posters intended to convey. What the slogan *does* say clearly is that parents have a "right" to comply with the government's recommendation to breastfeed exclusively. Needless to say, this slogan uses the word *right* in a way that turns the very concept of rights—as a vehicle of human empowerment and autonomy—on its head. It's the kind of line you might expect to find in a bad cop movie: "You have the right to do what we tell you to do."

THE WOMEN WHO WERE MOST INCENSED about Latch On NYC—who expressed outrage on television, were quoted in news articles, and blogged and commented about it online— were almost all middle-class white women. By and large these are women who enjoy and exercise a great deal of autonomy in their everyday lives and are not generally subjected to direct state control and intervention. But the experiences of lower income women are quite different. The US government has a long history of using coercive tactics to get poor women to conform to its mandates, and breastfeeding is no exception.

More than half the babies born every year in the United States receive benefits from the Special Supplemental Nutrition Program for Women, Infants, and Children (WIC). In 2014, a family of two qualified for WIC if their annual household income was under $29,101—185 percent of the US Poverty Income Guidelines. WIC is the most extensive food assistance program in the country for mothers and young children. WIC is also the front line of American breastfeeding advocacy. Public health officials and advocates have relied for the most part on education and advertising to persuade middle-class women to breastfeed. But they have much more direct and effective ways of targeting poor mothers who depend, or partly depend, on government assistance through WIC to feed their families.

WIC offers food vouchers (which it calls checks) to eligible pregnant and postpartum mothers, infants, and children up to the age of five. WIC checks specify a list of foods they can be used to purchase, and the checks can be redeemed at participating WIC stores. Stores that sell WIC products and participate in the WIC voucher scheme are common in poor neighborhoods, and they post signs on their shelves indicating that a particular product (this size and this brand, for example) is allowable under WIC. In some states there are WIC-only stores that sell nothing but WIC-approved products. The stores collect vouchers from customers and are then reimbursed through the WIC program.

WIC checks are precise about what food WIC clients can purchase, and WIC allocates a certain dollar amount for specific fruits and vegetables. Brown rice is okay but not white rice or organic rice. Organic fruits and vegetables are fine; organic milk is not. WIC checks may be used to buy sweet potatoes but not plain potatoes, peanut butter but not peanuts. Mothers can buy American, cheddar, and part-skim mozzarella cheese, but not white cheddar or whole-milk mozzarella. WIC rules also specify what brand mothers must purchase. For people who depend on WIC, shopping for food can be a complicated and time-consuming burden.

WIC was an early adopter of breastfeeding advocacy: it has been formally mandated to promote breastfeeding since its inception in 1974. But the organization renewed its attention to breastfeeding in the late 1980s, with new legislation that authorized a series of specific promotional activities starting in 1989. In 1994, Congress passed legislation requiring WIC state agencies to spend twenty-one dollars on breastfeeding promotion and support for each pregnant or breastfeeding woman who went through their offices. In 1997, the US Department of Agriculture (USDA) implemented the "Loving Support Makes Breastfeeding Work" campaign to increase breastfeeding rates among WIC mothers. Since 1998, WIC has been required to divert funds previously allocated for food to purchase breast pumps and hire lactation consultants and to provide breastfeeding education and support, including counseling and promotional materials.

In 2009, WIC took additional steps to "expand the scope of WIC's activities to encourage and support its participants in breastfeeding" by increasing federal oversight of WIC programs. The USDA, which administers WIC, promulgated a series of new regulations to ensure that WIC offices uniformly enforced the mandate to make breastfeeding its top priority. Among other things, it allowed WIC programs to divert more funding for food to breastfeeding support and advised WIC counselors to prioritize certification of breastfeeding mothers and children over nonbreastfeeding mothers and children. WIC is not an entitlement program, which means that it only serves clients up to the point that funding runs out. By prioritizing the certification of breastfeeding families, WIC was establishing nonbreastfeeding as a criterion for being turned away from WIC.

For me, the most outrageous feature of WIC's breastfeeding campaign was its 2009 decision to offer an "enhanced food package" to breastfeeding mothers and their infants. The enhanced food package allows breastfeeding mothers to stay on WIC for one year after their baby is born, whereas nonbreastfeeding mothers are eligible for only six months. The enhanced food package also promotes breastfeeding by offering "a food package of higher monetary value" with a "wider variety of better quality and more nutritious food" to breastfeeding mothers than to nonbreastfeeding mothers. Infants who are breastfed will also get more, and better, food than infants who are not breastfed.

WIC food allocations also distinguish between fully breastfeeding and partially breastfeeding mothers. Fully breastfeeding mothers get the widest variety of better quality and more nutritious food, partially breastfeeding mothers get less, and the "nonbreastfeeding food package" offers mothers "the least amount of foods." A mother who requests formula when her baby is less than one month old will receive the nonbreastfeeding food package, even if she is partially breastfeeding.

According to the promotional materials WIC gives to pregnant women and mothers seeking WIC assistance, "fully breastfeeding mothers will receive more milk, cheese, eggs, fruits, and vegetables, they do not have to choose between peanut butter and beans" (they can have both), and "they will also receive canned fish" (tuna fish, salmon, etc.). Women who are exclusively breastfeeding multiple infants (twins or triplets) get 1.5 times the "fully breastfeeding" food package. Babies who are fully breastfed are also eligible for more and better food. "As an incentive to encourage breastfeeding, fully breastfed infants will receive infant meats, in addition to an increased quantity of infant fruits and vegetables." Babies who are not exclusively breastfed get less baby food than fully breastfed babies, and their vouchers cover only fruit and vegetables, not meat.

WIC is clear that the reason it offers breastfeeding mothers more, and better, food is to provide "incentives for mothers to breastfeed without supplementation." WIC counselors are required, for example, to tell mothers that "around 6 months of age all babies need food that supplies iron and zinc. Meat is one of the best sources of these nutrients. As an incentive to encourage breastfeeding, fully breastfed infants will receive infant meats, in addition to an increased quantity of infant fruits and vegetables." After explaining what nutrients their babies need, WIC counselors are instructed to tell mothers that WIC will not provide those nutrients unless the mother breastfeeds exclusively.

WIC does not make exceptions to its policy of allocating food on the basis of breastfeeding status, even if a woman cannot breastfeed or has been instructed by her doctor to feed her baby formula or to supplement with formula. "No," explained the director of the WIC program for Western New York. "We don't make any exceptions. The mother must be breastfeeding to receive the breastfeeding food package."

Although WIC is a federally funded program, with formal policies and directives that come from its headquarters in Washington, DC, it is actually administered through a wide range of organizations. Hospitals have WIC programs and so do churches and community centers. State and city governments also have WIC programs, run out of state and city government buildings. In New York state, WIC centers are run through institutions as diverse as Catholic Charities of Western New York, the Bronx Lebanon Hospital Center, the Brownsville Community Development Corporation, and the Monroe County Health Department.

Ever since the enhanced food package went into effect, WIC enrollment has declined steadily, from 9.3 million in 2009 to fewer than 9 million in 2014. This decline is striking not only because enrollment in the SNAP/Food Stamp Program is at an all-time high, but also because eligibility for WIC is less restrictive. WIC women do not have to meet the same poverty threshold that SNAP recipients do.

WIC officials say they cannot explain the declining enrollment in their program, although they do worry about it. They are aware that declining enrollment is likely to mean budget cuts, and they know that, in fact, lots of families who don't enroll really need WIC.

But it really isn't that difficult to figure out why WIC enrollment is declining. Many mothers harbor deep resentment toward the program. For benefits that add up to about forty-seven dollars per month, the program makes them jump through hoops that many women find too time consuming to fit into their already punishing schedules. They have to requalify every six months. Every time they requalify, they have to take courses. Often it's the same course over and over again, usually on the

benefits of breastfeeding, even if the mother is not breastfeeding. It's difficult to figure out what you can and cannot buy with
your WIC checks. The food options are extremely limited. Store
cashiers and customers are often very rude to women paying
for groceries with WIC checks.

What women seem to resent most, however, is the way
many WIC employees and counselors treat them, especially
when it comes to breastfeeding. No doubt some offices make
a point of respecting a mother's decision to formula-feed her
infant. But many others seem to translate WIC's official breastfeeding mandate as a license to browbeat and humiliate women
into fulfilling WIC goals.

There are literally hundreds of comments online from
women complaining about how WIC counselors treat them.
The comments crop up on mainstream websites like Baby
Center, feminist websites like Jezebel and Feministe, and even
completely random websites like Yahoo! Answers. Joining one
conversation, a mother lamented, "I breastfed my daughter until she was 8 months (still do occasionally) but the whole time
i could only produce less than 2 or 3 ounces the whole day.
When i went to wic and told them they treated me like i was
a failure and stupid. They were very rude when I said I had to
supplement." Another mother chimed in with her own story.
"When I went into my first WIC appointment, I was breastfeeding and all was well. The next time I told them that my milk
was drying up and I needed to use formula, it felt like I had to
BEG them to put my baby on the formula program. I kinda felt
like a criminal asking for formula. You would think I wanted
to feed my baby poison or something." I spoke to two mothers
who had been enrolled in WIC when their babies were small,
one in Texas and one in Harlem. Both of them had quit WIC

before their eligibility ran out because the WIC counselors were so heavy-handed.

Posting on Feministe, which has followers on Facebook, Flickr, and Twitter, a mother who was on WIC explained: "In my experience, WIC is super-shamey, period. Before I could get my vouchers, I had to take anger-management classes on how not to beat my children (among other courses). These were mandated regardless of our parenting methods, history with children, record of violence or lack thereof, etc. It's really nice to be assumed to abuse your children because you need help paying for food." Another mother was berated for requesting a pump: the WIC counselor told her she had to be nursing, at the breast, to receive the enhanced food package. Another mother, who was under a doctor's instruction not to breastfeed, was forced to defend herself every time she picked up her vouchers. Another mother recalled that her WIC-mandated breastfeeding class was taught by an officer from Child Protection Services, which she took as a fairly direct warning that CPS was monitoring infant-feeding practices. Some reported being criticized for breastfeeding *too much*. "I got yelled at by wic over breastfeeding my son past a year and that is when I refused to get wic any more."

ALONG WITH POOR WOMEN, the US government's breastfeeding advocacy campaigns have also targeted African American women, even when they do not qualify for WIC. Through the National Immunization Survey, the Centers for Disease Control and Prevention (CDC) collects, and annually reports, breastfeeding data according to race, sex (of the child), birth order, mother's age, mother's education, mother's marital status, residence, poverty-income ratio, and whether or not the mother is enrolled in WIC. That data reveals that African American women lag behind white women in breastfeeding initiation and duration. When the results of that survey are released every year, and published on the CDC website, it is the message about racial differences that is most often picked up and reported by media outlets. In fact, employment status, which I discuss at greater length in Chapter 5, has a greater effect on breastfeeding rates, but is completely overlooked in the CDC's catalogue of "socio-demographic factors" that affect breastfeeding.

This way of reporting breastfeeding data has prompted the DHHS to target African Americans with specifically designed breastfeeding interventions. The CDC acknowledges that the racial gap has in fact narrowed significantly in recent years, to 15 percent among children born in 2010, but it nevertheless continues to insist that "more targeted strategies to increase breastfeeding support for African American mothers are still needed."

Most of these strategies are billed as educational. The main educational resource for African American women is called *An Easy Guide to Breastfeeding for African American Women.* The difference between this guide and publications designed for other populations is that it is extremely *easy.* While other publications make the case for breastfeeding by focusing on the scientific evidence of its benefits, *An Easy Guide* skips the scientific details. Readers are told only that "nursing mothers and most healthcare providers agree that the benefits of breastfeeding are endless." The guide also makes the incongruous claim, which I did not find in guides geared toward other population groups, that "breastfeeding mothers have more self-esteem." Finally, the guide warns that mothers living with HIV/AIDS and mothers who use "street drugs" should not breastfeed.

Breastfeeding advocacy campaigns also target African Americans. The national "Babies were born to be breastfed" campaign featured one radio ad in which a man with a heavy African American accent sang a soul song about breastfeeding to his girlfriend and baby. The gag was the intentional blurring of the word *baby*. The same campaign produced a television ad showing an extremely pregnant African American woman riding a mechanical bull in a bar. A neon sign above her head says "Ladies Night." Ultimately, the woman is thrown from the bull. The location, along with the woman's behavior, suggests she's been drinking. The screen reads "You wouldn't take risks before your baby is born. Why start after? Breastfeed exclusively for six months." A male voice-over describes the medical benefits of breastfeeding.

The goal of this campaign was to focus attention on the risks associated with formula feeding rather than the benefits of breastfeeding. The ad's not very subtle message was that feeding your baby formula is as risky as drinking and riding a mechanical bull when you are nine months pregnant. The ad sparked outrage among many women and prompted the AAP to withdraw support from the breastfeeding campaign. Critics argued that the ad was insulting to women, and they urged DHHS to focus attention instead on the structural barriers faced by women who want to breastfeed.

What is surprising, however, is that these critics did not mention the decision to portray the mechanical bull-riding woman as African American. This decision no doubt drew on, and certainly reinforced, the constantly cited evidence showing that African American women breastfeed less often than white women. But it also portrayed African Americans as especially prone to risk taking—the cartoonishly risky behavior featured in the ad standing in for the risks of formula feeding. Like so many other breastfeeding advocacy measures aimed at African American women, this one almost certainly failed to change the infant-feeding practices of the women it targeted. It did, however, succeed in reinforcing racial stereotypes about the substandard nature of African American parenting practices.

A few months after this ad aired, when I was pregnant with my first child in 2005, I was subjected to a somewhat surreal lecture on the benefits of breastfeeding at a party, the same one I mentioned in the introduction. When the lecturer got to the part about the appalling racial disparities in breastfeeding rates, she mentioned the mechanical bull ad as evidence that black women were making bad parenting decisions. Her description seemed to imply that the ad had filmed a true event, rather than staged a fake one. When I pointed out that the ad wasn't real, she brushed aside my objection: "Yeah, but it's the sort of thing that happens all the time." "What?" I blurted out, stunned. "Pregnant black women get drunk and ride mechanical bulls in bars all the time?! Seriously?" The woman replied that she had recently become a member of La Leche League and had been reading a lot of "research" that confirmed that the basic premise of the ad was in fact true.

What shocked me the most was that this woman was not obviously stupid or racist. OK, I take it back. Obviously she was both stupid and racist, but not ostensibly. A white upper-middle-class Democrat from Manhattan would not normally be caught dead revealing her prejudices. But she seemed to believe that her concerns about breastfeeding, not to mention the authority she had evidently garnered through her membership in La Leche League, gave her some kind of license to air opinions that were distinctly racist.

Breastfeeding advocates and public health officials will tell you, and may actually believe, that their "targeted" interventions are benevolent. They are billed as well-intentioned efforts to reduce racial inequities in breastfeeding, to ensure that the benefits of breastfeeding are experienced more broadly. But they are also ignorant and offensive. Race is actually not the most important factor in determining who does and doesn't breastfeed. Yet the many breastfeeding campaigns targeting African Americans reinforce racial stereotypes and send strong messages about which demographics parent best—and worst.

Comparatively low breastfeeding rates among African Americans have also generated targeted research to find out why black women avoid breastfeeding. Those studies routinely show that the overwhelming reason black women give for not breastfeeding is that they "prefer to bottle feed." They state a clear and simple preference against breastfeeding. Efforts to explain this preference have led the CDC to hypothesize that black women may "lack culturally relevant information," may hold "perceptions that breastfeeding is inferior to formula feeding," may "lack social or partner support," and "lack knowledge of the health benefits associated with breastfeeding." In other words, public health officials attribute African American mothers' preference for formula to their own misinformation, misperception, and ignorance and to the misinformation, misperception, and ignorance of their partners and community. They do not study why white women do not breastfeed.

Yet there is good reason to think that African American mothers' preference for formula feeding is not a product of ignorance. For one thing, although they have been repeatedly subjected to so-called educational campaigns for at least twenty years now, research shows that those campaigns have had little

effect. Even New York City's Latch On campaign, with its mandated talking-to's and multiple injunctions to educate mothers
on the benefits of breastfeeding, was mostly unsuccessful.

In *At the Breast*, an excellent and well-researched book on
breastfeeding in the United States, the author and sociologist
Linda Blum shows that many African American mothers prefer formula feeding for a complex range of reasons. They tend
to share parenting responsibilities with a network of relatives
and friends. Breastfeeding, they feel, is more suited to a model
of exclusive mothering they neither practice nor believe in.
Blum also found that the demands of the workplace make
breastfeeding difficult for African Americans in much the
same way they do for other working-class women. According
to Blum, "concerns with negotiating workplace, school, and
hectic households, and with their over-work as working class
mothers, played a major role in the Black mothers' rejection
of breastfeeding." In the interviews Blum conducted, African
American mothers also expressed concerns about violations
of privacy and respectability involved with breastfeeding in
public and with pumping.

When Blum asked her interviewees explicitly whether they
were aware of the benefits associated with breastfeeding, most
laughed and rolled their eyes, telling her things like, "It's all anyone ever talked about," and "I would get pamphlets every time I
went to the doctor." Every one of the African American women
she interviewed had heard that "breast is best," and many even
believed it. But for other reasons, they still held distinct preferences to feed their babies formula.

Against the backdrop of strained and highly politicized racial relations, in a country that has been wracked with virulent
racism from its very inception, it is hard to believe that policy

makers do not realize the effect of their continued and insistent emphasis on African Americans' "conspicuously lower" rates of breastfeeding. Especially when they insist on framing breast-feeding as a civic responsibility, a way mothers can save money for all Americans and contribute to the health of the nation, the focus on African American infant-feeding practices seems al-most *designed* to fuel American race wars and to remind white Americans that, after all, they really *are* better parents and bet-ter citizens.

SINCE AT LEAST THE FIRST CLINTON administration, when Hil-lary Clinton's effort to reform the American health-care system failed, health care has been the most pressing domestic prob-lem in the United States. Annual health-care expenditure in the US is $2.6 trillion. The American health-care industry is larger than the economy of France. Meanwhile the cost of health care is soaring. Between 1999 and 2010, the cost of health insurance increased 131 percent. A 2012 poll revealed that 28 percent of middle-income families were having a serious problem paying for health care or health insurance. Even after the Affordable Care Act extended insurance to twenty million people, 13.4 percent of Americans were still uninsured in 2014, and the ACA has not tackled one of the crisis's most basic problems: the exorbitant cost of health care in the US.

Faced with this seemingly intractable crisis, politicians, pol-icy makers, and public health officials have begun to insist that our health-care problems are a matter of individual responsi-bility. This shift has been accompanied by a new emphasis on chronic illnesses. The CDC reports that "75% of total health care spending in the United States goes towards the treatment of chronic diseases, such as diabetes and asthma." Chronic diseases are, in turn, defined as those that are caused or aggravated by the afflicted individuals themselves. The DHHS and the CDC consistently emphasize the same four themes: chronic diseases are the leading cause of death and disability in the United States; chronic diseases are responsible for soaring health-care costs and an overwhelmed health-care system; chronic diseases are particularly costly for employers; and chronic diseases are mostly preventable "through simple life-style changes."

For many years, smoking and unsafe sex dominated public and official perceptions of the individual lifestyle choices that threatened public health. Lung diseases, some types of cancer, herpes, and HIV/AIDS could all be traced to so-called lifestyle choices like smoking and unsafe sex. Large education and advertising campaigns, as well as smoking bans, "sin" taxes on cigarette sales, advertising regulations, and crackdowns on bathhouses and prostitution were initiated to combat these threats to public health.

In the late 1990s, obesity was added to the roster of leading preventable causes of chronic disease. In 1997, the World Health Organization identified obesity as a "global epidemic," and the CDC dates the start of the American "obesity epidemic" to the late 1990s. The surgeon general, the CDC, and DHHS also began to focus significant attention on obesity in the second half of the 2000s, initiating various campaigns and calls to action. In January 2013 ScienceDaily published an article titled "Obesity Approaching Cigarette Smoking as Leading Avoidable Cause of Premature Deaths," and a 2013 WebMD featured article quoted a nutritionist saying "at the rate we're going, obesity-related diabetes alone will break the bank of our healthcare system." In the same year, the American Medical Association took the significant step of identifying obesity as a disease.

By officially designating breastfeeding as a public health is-sue, the surgeon general, the CDC, DHHS, and the AAP have now placed formula feeding alongside other irresponsible life-style choices that are overburdening the US health-care sys-tem—just like unsafe sex, smoking, and unhealthy eating.

In 1975, the *Chicago Tribune* opined that "the idea of pre-ventive medicine is faintly un-American. It means, first, recog-nizing that the enemy is us." From my perspective, this gets it exactly backward. Preventive medicine strikes me as a *distinctly* American approach to health and illness precisely because it attributes primary responsibility for health outcomes to indi-vidual behavior. The prevention doctrine merely extends the Horatio Alger story, the story of the American dream pursued and achieved through hard work and moral fortitude, from the realm of economics to the realm of physical health. As our health policy organizations focus increasing attention on "indi-vidual lifestyle choices" as the primary cause of illness in Amer-ica, they drive home the message that whether we succeed or fail at being healthy is our own responsibility.

By blaming individual lifestyle choices for the crisis of American health care, policy makers are, of course, also trans-ferring responsibility for health outcomes from health-care providers, insurance companies, and the US government to in-dividual citizens. At the same time, they are offering a magic bullet solution to a complex and intractable problem: if only Americans ate fewer fries and more fiber, the health-care crisis, including soaring costs, corrupt billing practices, and millions of still uninsured Americans, would be solved.

People will disagree over the appropriateness of public health initiatives. Is it appropriate for the government to try to influ-ence citizens' behavior? And, if so, where do you draw the line between legitimate interventions and overstepping? Because of his many public health initiatives, Mayor Bloomberg was often criticized for running a "nanny state" in New York City. Even people who agree that the government should play some role in encouraging people to adopt a healthier lifestyle will disagree over what issues legitimately count as public health issues: Is formula feeding really the same as smoking?

They will also disagree over how far the government should go to do that: Is it OK to penalize poor women who don't breastfeed by denying them the same number and caliber of benefits provided to women who do? They may also disagree about who the appropriate object for public health initiatives is: Should we be concerned when coercive tactics designed to influence individual behavior overwhelmingly target a particular segment of the population? These questions highlight the ways in which breastfeeding advocacy can descend into lactivism, adopting more or less coercive measures depending on the population they target. Not one of the public breastfeeding initiatives launched since 1995 seems directed toward supporting women's own preferences and choices.

CHAPTER 5

Pumping on the Job

When Abigail Reed, a successful advertising executive in San Francisco with a go-get-'em attitude, went back to work six weeks after her first child was born, she fully expected to keep breastfeeding her baby for at least six months. She found a small, out-of-the-way storage room at her office where she sequestered herself three times a day, pumping for about thirty minutes each time.

Often, though, she had to attend meetings when she should have been pumping. When she had to skip those pumping sessions, her breast milk leaked, and twice it leaked through her bra and nursing pads, staining her silk shirt. The second time that happened, her younger female boss carefully reminded Reed of the importance of professionalism in the workplace. After the second week, Reed's milk supply started to diminish because she wasn't pumping frequently enough. Her nanny started to supplement fresh breast milk with frozen breast milk, and then with formula.

In her fourth week back at work, Reed was scheduled to lead an all-day sales pitch at the company of a big potential client in the food industry. The company was an hour away from Reed's office in San Francisco, and they would be in meetings with different teams all day long. As she prepared for the meeting, Reed realized she would not be able to duck out to pump that day. Her breasts would become engorged, which would be excruciating and might even lead to mastitis. But worse still, from Reed's perspective, there was a chance she might leak. She was the lead person on the account. She and her team had worked on it for months. She had no choice but to attend the meeting, and she couldn't risk any sort of "unprofessionalism" that might compromise their sales pitch.

Reed felt increasingly trapped. Three weeks after returning from maternity leave, her son now nine weeks old, she realized she had to choose between work and breastfeeding. Even though she had a good job and was legally entitled to pump at work, the practical demands of her work schedule made it impossible. Miserable and plagued by feelings of guilt and failure, she stopped breastfeeding. When her second son was born, Reed quit her job to stay at home with her children.

REED'S EXPERIENCE IS JUST ONE EXAMPLE of how hard it can be, even for women in relatively privileged jobs, to combine breastfeeding and work. Well-paid professional women who pump at work frequently report having a very difficult time maintaining their hard-won authority and respect in the office while managing an uncompromising work schedule. One friend of mine who held a senior position in a tech company told me that young men in her office, who had treated her with the deference due to her status before she had a baby, developed a habit of making snide comments when she walked past them on her way to pump breast milk. She was humiliated. Not long after, she quit. Women who work as teachers, hospital doctors, nurses, or in the service sector as, say, store clerks or waitresses, often report that pumping at work is not just difficult but impossible. Either there is no space or no time, or both.

Nevertheless, the US government's recent initiatives to promote breastfeeding have focused almost exclusively on breast pumping. Most of these campaigns have been launched with great fanfare and publicity, and they have been lauded as supportive of breastfeeding and women. But, without even acknowledging this important shift from breast to pump, they have radically redefined what breastfeeding is. To be clear, pumping at work can help a mother maintain her milk supply so that she can also nurse her baby at home on weekends or in the evening. But the government's recent so-called breastfeeding initiatives are designed to help a woman pump breast milk at work so that someone else can feed her baby breast milk from a bottle. In other words, these much-vaunted initiatives depend on the unstated—and largely unstudied—premise that what is valuable about breastfeeding is the chemical composition of human milk, *not* the mother-child contact that goes along with feeding a baby at the breast.

That premise is a long way from the set of beliefs that initially motivated the founding mothers of La Leche League, who believed that the benefits of breastfeeding came primarily from the intimacy of nursing. It is also a long way from the attachment parenting philosophy promoted by Dr. Sears and others, who see breastfeeding as an important way to develop a strong mother-child bond.

Pumping breast milk is also a peculiarly American form of "breastfeeding." Nowhere else in the world, including in other developed countries, do women use breast pumps as much as they do in the United States. Most American mothers say they pump so they can return to their jobs. And in fact it's clear that pumping has emerged as a widely adopted work-around that allows women to return to their jobs without depriving their babies of the now accepted benefits of "breastfeeding."

Public health campaigns that promote pumping are thus quietly overturning the expectation that breastfeeding depends, first and foremost, on direct contact between a mother and her baby. By upending that expectation, policy makers build an effective defense against arguments for paid federally mandated maternity leave. Who needs a lavish European-style maternity leave when a mother's body is no longer the only vehicle through which the magic elixir, mother's milk, can be delivered? Such campaigns have also transformed breastfeeding, which was once seen as a challenge against big business, into big business itself. By 2020, the US market for breast pumps will reach almost $1 billion, and the related market for breastfeeding and pumping accessories will be roughly double that.

MANY WOMEN LOVE BREASTFEEDING. They may enjoy watching their babies nuzzle at the breast, making little noises of contentment while they eat. They may even get the famous endorphin rush, an almost Zen-like feeling of peace and contentment that some lucky women have experienced. Breastfeeding puts some women in touch with their "inner earth mother," and they derive deep satisfaction from the fact that what their baby needs most is *them*.

I'll admit that I never found the experience of breastfeeding transporting or magical, and I certainly never experienced any endorphin high. But I did love the way it quickly comforted and calmed my babies when they were hurt or upset. If breastfeeding does come easily to you and your baby, it is extremely convenient, and not just for feeding. There's probably nothing like breastfeeding to comfort a baby after a vaccination—or a fall, or a very long day. Even in the face of evidence that breastfeeding does not offer many of the health benefits attributed to it, lots of women would no doubt still choose to breastfeed just because it works for them and their babies.

Pumping, however, is a different story altogether. I will bet there isn't a woman alive who loves pumping. Pumping sucks—and that's not just a bad pun. Both electric and manual pumps have a see-through breast shield or flange, which is placed over the nipple. The transparent shield enables you to watch your nipple being yanked and elongated with every compression, as the milk funnels into a plastic bottle attached to the shield. If you have a manual pump, which costs about forty dollars, you hold the shield on your breast with one hand while the other squeezes a plastic pump over and over. It's tricky to manage, and difficult to extract enough milk to feed a baby. Electric pumps are less portable than manual ones but much easier to use, since they do the pumping for you, and are also much more efficient. The newer double pumps are even more efficient. They feature twin shields and bottles that enable mothers to drain both breasts at once. Some of the latest models are even hands-free. The shields are attached to a bra, making it possible to talk on the phone, or maybe even cook dinner, while pumping. *Ta-da!*

An instructional video sponsored by the company that makes the Hands Free Pump Bra demonstrates how to set up and use the hands-free pump. (Actually, there are lots of pumping videos online, but most of them seem most likely to be watched by men and are not very "instructional.") The video's perky female voice instructs the user to "slip in your breast pump horns." Meanwhile the video, depicting only a woman's torso, no head, shows her slipping clear plastic cylinders (the horns) through small openings in the pump bra and then fitting the shields, which are attached to the horns, on her nipples.

For the first few months especially, mothers are advised to empty their breasts each time they pump to build up and maintain their milk supply. That process can easily take up to about thirty minutes per breast, which is why the double pump is a good investment. After the milk has been expressed, each part of the pump has to be cleaned and sterilized so that old milk is not left on the sides of the tubes and suction cups. Then the milk needs to be labeled and safely stored. For someone lucky enough to be in possession of a double pump, the whole process might take about forty-five minutes. In the course of an eight-hour work day, a mother would have to do this two or three times, depending on the age of the baby and how often he eats.

So why don't women like pumping? For most women it's uncomfortable, and some find it painful. All that pulling and yanking hurts. Some moms have had their nipples ripped to shreds. On an admittedly more minor note, several women report that the noise of the pump and the sucking sound drives them crazy, especially in the middle of the night. Almost everyone complains that pumping takes up so much time—and that it's boring. With a hands-free pump, you can, in theory, take conference calls, as the chief operating officer of Facebook, Sheryl Sandberg, claims to have done in her book *Lean In*. But even Sandberg had to cover for herself by telling colleagues and clients that the beeping sounds her pump made were coming from a passing fire engine. Lots of women say they drive to work while using a hands-free pump, which saves them time, but doesn't seem very safe. If talking on your cell phone is illegal, surely pumping and driving should be illegal too. Still, pumping and driving is common enough that stores that sell pumping equipment and accessories usually sell car adapters too.

For the most part, however, it is really difficult to go about your normal routine with horns and bottles hanging off your breasts. You can't go outside, and you really shouldn't have people over. It's also very hard to type. You can't answer the door, and you should probably resist the urge to plant bulbs in your garden. In general it's best not to *lean in* too far when there are horns and bottles dangling from your boobs. First and foremost, however, women do not like pumping because they experience it as humiliating and degrading, especially when they are forced to do it at work, usually in cramped spaces and rushed situations.

But, even though they don't like it, and may actively *dislike* it, most American women who breastfeed also pump. One study found that 85 percent of women with babies younger than four and a half months had expressed milk. Medela, one of the leading manufacturers of breast pumps and pumping equipment in the world, claims that somewhere between 80 and 90 percent of breastfeeding mothers in the US use a pump. Amanda Cole, the owner of Yummy Mummy, estimates that "basically everyone" uses a pump. Older mothers in a higher income bracket are more likely to pump than poorer and younger mothers. Twenty-five percent of breastfeeding mothers are on a regular pumping schedule. These women are more than likely employed. Most women who pump say they do it to get breast milk for someone else to feed their baby while they are at work.

These percentages translate into fairly high numbers of women. In 2012, almost 4 million (3,952,841) babies were born in the United States. Seventy-nine percent (3.1 million) start breastfeeding, and forty-nine percent (1.94 million) are still breastfeeding at six months. This means that in 2012, 2.6 million women in the US used a breast pump at least occasionally, and between half a million and 775,000 women used a breast pump routinely.

One apparently small subset of lactating women—roughly 6 percent—identify themselves as exclusive pumpers, EPs for short. The number of EPs is high enough that almost every breastfeeding or parenting website has a section devoted to exclusive pumping, and EPs have at least one dedicated website. The website's home page welcomes visitors "to the wacky world of exclusively pumping." It features an image of a woman pumping while driving, the horns sticking out from under her shirt. With evident pride, the enthusiastic caption above the image exclaims, "We Pump Everywhere!"

Exclusive pumping takes the importance of human milk more or less for granted. Why do people exclusively pump? the site asks. "Because we feel breastmilk is best even in a bottle." For any number of reasons, these women are unable to breastfeed, but able to pump. The website is a support group for women who are feeling isolated because they are not really breastfeeding in the traditional sense of the word, but neither are they formula feeding. It supports their choice to exclusively pump—a choice that, they say, seems crazy to most people. But they do it because they believe in the benefits of human milk, regardless of how it is delivered.

SINCE 2001, THE ANNUAL National Immunization Survey has collected data on breastfeeding. As I mentioned in the last chapter, when the CDC compiles and publishes that data, it breaks down breastfeeding rates by state, race, and socioeconomic and marital status. But it does not record differences in breastfeeding initiation and duration based on employment status. This is a significant omission since employment is one of the most important factors in determining whether and how long American women breastfeed. In fact, a 2006 study showed that mothers who don't work are more than twice as likely to be breastfeeding at six months than mothers who work full-time. An earlier study, published in 1998, also found that mothers who expected to return to work were less likely to initiate breastfeeding at all. Whereas 81.5 percent of mothers who did not plan to work postpartum initiated breastfeeding, only 67.2 percent of those who did intend to work full-time initiated breastfeeding. Working women are 14 percent less likely to start breastfeeding than nonworking women.

That same study also found that employment has a notable impact on how long women breastfeed. "Full-time working mothers breastfed an average of 16.5 weeks, which was 8.6 less than non-working mothers." Nonworking mothers, in other words, breastfeed an average of 25.1 weeks, which is basically six months. Nonworking mothers meet national breastfeeding goals, and working mothers do not. A more recent study from 2011 reported, similarly, that 47 percent of women who don't work are still breastfeeding at six months, compared with only 30 percent of women who return to work before three months.

That 17 percent difference is higher than the constantly cited difference between black and white women, which was 15 percent in 2010. What it reveals is that employment status is at least as important as race in determining breastfeeding initiation and duration. Yet employment is remarkably, even shockingly, absent from our public conversations about breastfeeding. An online search will uncover only three articles, all cited above, on employment and breastfeeding in the United States. Yet every single policy and reporting document, as well as the data and statistics released annually by the CDC, mentions racial breastfeeding disparities, and there are literally hundreds of articles describing and analyzing the problem of racial disparities in breastfeeding.

It's hard to resist the conclusion that the reason public health initiatives and policy makers don't discuss the effect of maternal employment on breastfeeding rates is that doing so would focus attention squarely on America's famously skimpy maternity leave. The United States is the only developed country in the world with no mandatory paid maternity leave. In fact it is one of only 4 countries—out of a total 173—with no national policy requiring paid maternity leave. The others are Swaziland, Liberia, and Papua New Guinea. For the 71 percent of American mothers who work outside the home, paid maternity leave would undoubtedly make six months of exclusive breastfeeding not just more attractive but possible. Yet such a policy is not even on the table.

Instead, "approximately 14% of US employers offer paid maternity leave beyond short-term disability benefits." *The Surgeon General's Call to Action to Support Breastfeeding* reports, not surprisingly, that higher paid employees are more likely to have this benefit. Fourteen percent of management and professional workers have this benefit, while only 4 percent of industrial workers have it. Only 5 percent of employees who earn less than fifteen dollars an hour have any paid maternity leave whatsoever.

Most women in the United States are allowed twelve weeks of unpaid leave around the birth or adoption of a baby. For many mothers, however, it is financially impossible to take twelve weeks of leave without pay. And if a mother works for a company with fewer than fifty employees, or has worked there for less than one year, or is among the top 10 percent of earners in the company, the employer is not obligated to give her even those twelve weeks of unpaid leave. Some women are able to cobble together a paid or partly paid maternity leave by using a combination of short-term disability, sick leave, vacation, and personal days. The American Pregnancy Association warns families to plan carefully to avoid financial hardship. On average, women in the United States take six weeks of maternity leave, but fully 30 percent of women report that they take *no maternity leave at all*. That number also differs by race: 40 percent of Hispanic women, 31 percent of African American women, and 27 percent of white women take no maternity leave.

Between 2010 and 2013, President Obama presided over three breastfeeding initiatives. These efforts earned him effusive praise from breastfeeding advocates, women's organizations, and the medical community. What nobody seemed to notice, however, was that every single one of his initiatives was designed to promote pumping, not breastfeeding as it has been traditionally defined. Obama's pumping policies compel mothers to square the circle between the absence of maternity leave and the injunction to breastfeed exclusively for six months by pumping breast milk at work.

Obama's first initiative, launched in 2010 as part of the Affordable Care Act (ACA), amended the Fair Labor Standards Act to compel employers to "provide reasonable break time" for an employee to express milk for her child's first twelve months. On the face of it, this law seems designed to safeguard the rights of employees. That is certainly how the law has been sold—not only by Obama but also by breastfeeding advocates. But the fact remains that the law makes so many concessions to employers that it is far less worker- or mother-friendly than it sounds.

One of this law's important but rarely discussed limitations is that it allows employers to dock women for the time they spend pumping. "The employer is not required to compensate an employee receiving reasonable break time for any work time spent for such purpose." This means that many women who pump at work will need to take a pay cut. Employers are also allowed to require women to work longer hours to make up for the time they spend pumping during the day. In fact, the Department of Health and Human Services recommends that employers ask employees to come in early or stay late to make up the time they spend pumping breast milk. With a new baby at home, eight-hour workdays can easily stretch into nine- or ten-hour workdays.

The ACA regulation also offers a big loophole to small businesses by relieving them of any responsibility to support employees who need to pump at work: "If these requirements impose undue hardship, an employer that employs fewer than 50 employees is not subject to these requirements." Never mind imposing any undue hardship on the mother compelled to pump breast milk at work; the concern here is that small business owners should not have to bear any cost associated with breastfeeding.

The regulation's insistence that employers "must also provide a place, other than a bathroom, for the employee to express breast milk" has also turned out to be hopelessly vague. You would be shocked at the places employers routinely offer, including other peoples' offices, copier rooms, file rooms, broom closets, rooms made almost entirely of glass, and open

conference rooms. In a publication designed for business managers, the Department of Health and Human Services assures
business owners that the room can be as small as four by five
feet and recommends that they offer employees a closet or storage area if they have space constraints.

Many mothers report that pumping at work is stressful
because they live in constant fear of coworkers walking in on
them. Many say that coworkers have in fact walked in on them,
and there are a surprising number of news stories about women
being spied on by coworkers. A couple of women even discovered that their coworkers had videotaped them while they were
breast pumping: male coworkers had installed hidden cameras
in the rooms they used to pump. Presumably other women have
been videotaped but never discovered it. To avoid some of these
risks, many working mothers pump while they are driving to
work—abandoning privacy, modesty, and even safety in sheer
desperation.

BOBBI BOCKORAS WORKED AT A glass packaging factory in Port
Allegany, Pennsylvania. In April 2013, her daughter, Lyla, was
born. About a week after Lyla's birth, Bockoras texted her boss
to tell him she planned to pump when she returned to work so
that she could continue to breastfeed her baby. He told her she
could use the bathroom, and she advised him that a bathroom
was expressly prohibited by the ACA regulation. After this exchange she called the human resources manager to explain
what workplace accommodations she was entitled to under the
Nursing Mothers Provision.

Bockoras went back to work in mid-June, roughly six
weeks after Lyla was born. She was reassigned from her usual
job, which involved heavy lifting in confined spaces, to a less

physically demanding job. She was also told she could use the first-aid room to pump during her breaks, and she was put on the day shift. Bockoras was relieved that her managers seemed so responsive to her needs as a nursing mother.

Bockoras was one of only 30 women, however, out of a total workforce of 230, working at the glass factory. When she returned to work, she learned that her coworkers had joked that she would be pumping in the "cooling booth," an all-glass room where factory workers took breaks from the extreme heat of the factory floor. They had hung a sign in the booth that said "pump house." A coworker gave her a red bucket and made comments about milking a cow. These jokes made Bockoras self-conscious.

And they didn't stop. Men regularly banged on the first-aid room door when she was in there pumping, demanding to be let in. Bockoras sometimes worried they would break through. But when she complained to her boss that she was being harassed, he denied it and suggested some other places she could use. The first was a conference room with several large uncovered windows and two doors without locks. The second was a shower. The third was an unused locker room.

Bockoras chose the third option because it had a door she could lock. But the room was filthy. The floor was covered with dirt and dead bugs, and sections of the flooring were missing. A few days later, the only piece of furniture in the room, a chair, was removed. Her break wasn't long enough for her to go in search of another chair, so Bockoras sat down on the floor to pump. After her break, she complained about the missing chair to the human resources manager.

Later that same day, Bockoras was advised she would be switched from the day shift to the rotating day/night shift. She explained that a rotating schedule would interfere with her breastfeeding routine, and she submitted a doctor's note providing medical documentation. Other workers at the plant had often been given schedules that accommodated specific medical conditions, but in her case management refused to budge.

Meanwhile, pumping in the locker room got even worse. Male coworkers routinely banged on the metal door when she was in there. One day, someone covered the door handle with grease and sharp metal shards—a common prank at the factory. She reported the incident to her boss, and then it happened again. Her own union organizer made a lunchroom announcement that people should watch out for her because she had a lawyer and was "going after people for sexual harassment." After two months of this near-constant stress, coupled with the stress of the rotating day/night shifts, Bockoras's milk supply dropped by half. As her milk supply dwindled, Bockoras's baby began refusing to nurse.

Bobbi Bockoras's story is probably worse than most, but it's not unusual. In fact, the La Leche League web forum on working and breastfeeding is filled with miserable accounts of women's experiences pumping breast milk at work. Even women who have done it successfully admit that it is unpleasant—a sacrifice they are proud to have made for their children but a significant sacrifice nevertheless. Even the EPs are clear that pumping is a big burden.

Many working mothers have reported that they endure harassment from fellow employees who resent the time they spend pumping or who may have to fill in for them during a pumping break. One of the most common complaints of pumping mothers is that coworkers protest when mothers store their pumped milk in a communal refrigerator, allegedly fearful that her "bodily fluids" will contaminate their food. Almost every woman I have spoken to about pumping at work has at least one nasty or embarrassing story to tell, and they admit that pointed or derisive comments from coworkers, often masked as jokes, are common. But jokes about pumping breast milk at work deeply compromise a woman's dignity and professionalism and deserve to be taken seriously. It is hard to see how they don't constitute a form of harassment.

Still, Obama's reforms, combined with widespread support for breastfeeding, have made pumping at work seem like the new normal. Whereas not long ago breastfeeding and full-time employment were considered to be mutually exclusive—a woman can do one *or* the other—Obama's pro-pumping legislation has instead made it seem as if women can do both, at least if we are willing to accept the assumption that having someone else bottle-feed your baby expressed breast milk counts as breastfeeding. Pumping breast milk at work is something we have come to expect of new mothers. Now that women have the "right" to pump breast milk at work, "breastfeeding" appears to be perfectly compatible with a full-time job. As the Department of Health and Human Services crows, "Mothers do *not* have to choose between providing human milk for their baby and returning to work, and employers can retain valuable employees!" This apparent win-win solution enables women to "breastfeed" by working longer hours, for less pay, under conditions that are humiliating and degrading. Talk about "having it all."

And remarkably, even this woefully inadequate solution to the work/breastfeeding conflict often goes unenforced. Obama's much-celebrated amendment to the Fair Labor Act is toothless. Notwithstanding its stern pronouncement that "employers are not allowed to discriminate or retaliate against a woman who receives these accommodations," the law has no enforcement mechanism and offers no sanction against employers who violate the law. A few mothers have learned this the hard way, by initiating legal action.

The US Department of Labor Wage and Hour Division is ostensibly responsible for enforcing the law. But the department decided against issuing enforcement regulations because it wanted the regulation to be flexible around how many breaks a nursing mother might require and how employers might try to comply with the break-time requirement. The department says it prefers to address complaints on a case-by-case basis. Between March 2010, when the law went into effect, and January 2014, the department investigated 169 complaints and found 71 violations. But the law includes no penalty for businesses that fail to comply. The department can mediate between an employer and employee, and it can explain to the employer what its obligations are. But it cannot levy any fine against an employer for failing to comply. A small number of women have tried to take their employers to court for failing to comply with the regulation, but so far they have made little progress.

Angela Ames worked for Nationwide Mutual Insurance Company as a loss-mitigation specialist. Her baby was born on May 18, 2010, five weeks premature. Although Ames's boss told her initially that she could return to work on August 2, she later insisted that Ames return two weeks earlier, on July 19. When she got to work on the nineteenth, Ames told her department head she needed a place to pump. The department head responded that finding employees places to pump "was not her job" and referred her to the company nurse. The nurse told Ames she could not use the company's lactation rooms (even though there was one on every floor) because she first needed to fill out paperwork that would take three days to process.

Instead, she offered Ames a room where sick employees often rested, but warned that it would expose her to germs. At any rate, that room was being used by another employee who didn't feel well, and it had no lock on the door. Ames was told to check back in fifteen or twenty minutes. By this time her breasts were painfully engorged. When she returned in desperation to her boss, she told her to "just go home to be with your baby." Then she handed Ames a piece of paper and told her to write her own resignation letter. In tears, Ames did.

Some months later, Ames filed a discrimination complaint with the Iowa Civil Rights Commission. When that went nowhere, she sued Nationwide in 2012, alleging sex and pregnancy discrimination. Her claim was supported by the US Equal Employment Opportunity Commission (EEOC)—the government agency responsible for enforcing federal antidiscrimination laws. According to the EEOC, the relevant legal question was whether Title VII of the Civil Rights Act protects women from discrimination based on the stereotype that they would or should prefer to stay at home with their children. The EEOC thought that it did, and they filed a friend-of-the-court brief arguing that Ames had been a victim of discrimination. The lawsuit was dismissed by US District Judge Robert Pratt, of the Southern District of Iowa, however, who concluded "that no reasonable person would have found her working condition intolerable."

Again with backing from the EEOC, as well as the American Civil Liberties Union, Ames appealed that decision. But in March 2014, a federal appeals panel made up of three Republican-appointed men rejected Angela's request for a hearing. The somewhat incredible reasoning behind their decision was that "Nationwide's several attempts to accommodate Ames show its intent to maintain an employment relationship with Ames, not force her to quit." In June 2014, the Eighth Circuit Court of Appeal again denied Ames's request for a hearing. Even with the support of the EEOC, Ames was not even given a chance to tell her story in court.

On its face, the ACA regulation obliging employers to provide women the time and space necessary to express breast milk at work seems like a major advance for working women. But the reality is complicated, to say the least. What women are in fact offered is a lousy law that says they are now able to satisfy the mandate to "breastfeed" exclusively for six months while also returning to work. When that law is routinely violated, they are forced to fight for their "right" to pump at work. And when they take their employers to court for failing to comply with their legal obligations, judges have consistently sided with employers. In the end, the law sets up a whole new set of social expectations and norms for new mothers by creating the impression that they can, and should, pump at work. But mothers routinely find themselves unable to comply with those expectations both because of obstacles in the workplace and the government's failure to enforce the regulation.

Obama's second breastfeeding initiative was a tax deduction. In 2011, the IRS amended its policy to make breast-pumping equipment tax deductible, albeit only for taxpayers whose total medical expenses exceed 7.5 percent of their adjusted gross income. To be clear, that does not mean the government is paying for the pump, as Michele Bachmann so vociferously, but obtusely, complained. In fact, allowing parents to itemize and deduct the cost of a pump on their tax returns offers real savings only to parents in the highest tax brackets. For people in the lowest tax bracket, the tax deduction might reduce the cost of a $300 pump to $270, for a total savings of $30. But most people in the lowest tax brackets don't itemize deductions anyway; they're better off taking the standard deduction.

The tax deduction initiative was superseded in 2013, when the ACA mandated that private health insurance plans and Medicaid must cover the cost of breast pumps and other breast-feeding and breast-pumping support and equipment. Suddenly, every new mother in the United States was entitled to receive a free pump from her insurance company.

In 2015, journalist Steven Brill published a remarkable 455-page book describing the political and economic interests behind the passage of the Affordable Care Act. Every company that stood to gain from health-care reform had lobbyists running all over Capitol Hill. When I asked him about how free breast pumps had made it into the legislation, he said he had not heard specifically of a breast-pump manufacturers' lobby, but he would be surprised if they didn't have one.

I didn't find any evidence of such a lobby either, but breast-pump manufacturers certainly had a close ally in the Democratic senator from Maryland, Barbara Mikulski. Mikulski authored, and campaigned for the passage of, the Women's Health Amendment to the ACA, which included not only free breast pumps but free annual mammograms and contraception. According to Brill, the companies that make mammography equipment were well represented by lobbyists in Washington.

What free breast pumps mean in practice is still open to some interpretation, however. Breast pumps vary widely in price. Hand pumps cost between $40 and $50, but electric pumps cost between $300 and $400. Babies R Us sells the hospital-grade Medela Symphony pump for $2,224.99. Some insurance companies were not required to start coverage immediately for patients who were on older plans. New patients were eligible for the benefit in August 2012, others not until January 2013, and some even later than that.

Most insurance companies are covering or reimbursing the cost of a stripped-down version of an electric double-breast pump. This model allows women to pump both breasts at once, and it has a high-grade motor for good suctioning power, but it does not include all the accessories you could buy in a retail store. The insurance version doesn't include a cooler bag or a battery pack, and the carrying case is not as nice. Whereas the most popular pumps that include all the accessories cost around $400, the insurance pumps cost about $250.

After the ACA regulation went into effect, Medela repackaged its best-selling Pump In Style to meet the specifications of insurance companies. Now mothers can get the Pump In Style Advanced Breastpump Starter Set through their insurance company (it is not sold retail), and then purchase additional components separately. Medela also expanded the range of accessories that go with this pump, which mothers can buy in retail stores.

The pump reimbursement regulation ignited the already expanding market in breast pumps and related equipment. The United States has long represented the largest share of the global breast pump market, with about 40 percent of the world market share. In 2010, Medela claimed that the US breast pump market was 2.29 million units, including both manual and electric pumps. The ACA regulation not only expanded the US market for breast pumps, it also transformed it by practically eliminating demand for hand pumps (which really only work for the occasional emergency) and increasing the demand for much more expensive electric pumps. After January 2013, the demand for electric pumps increased by 50 percent, and suppliers struggled to keep up. Companies like Medela and Philips Avent, the two largest producers of breast pumps, quickly stepped up production.

The US market for breast pumps should eventually stabilize at about 3.5 million units per year—somewhere just below the number of annual live births in the US. If almost all pumps are sold through insurance companies at a cost of about $250, the US breast-pump market will be about $875 million. By 2015, the worldwide market is predicted to be just over $1.4 billion.

The subtle shift from breastfeeding to breast pumping has been a boon to the corporate fortunes of the companies that make breast pumps, like Ameda, Medela, Philips Avent, and Lansinoh. It also offers a good solution to employers who want to retain employees without paying the cost of maternity leave or absorbing the cost of the time a new mother spends breast-feeding. Pumping at work also offers a good solution to politicians who are loathe to propose regulations or legislation, like maternity leave, that might impose a cost on business, or that could be construed as a threat to the competitiveness of the American economy. It seems that the only losers in this win-win-win scenario are mothers and babies.

CHAPTER 6

Liquid Gold

Mother's milk soap calls for seventeen ounces of olive oil, eighteen ounces of safflower oil, two tablespoons of honey, and six cups of breast milk. Breast-milk ice cream uses only half a cup of breast milk, along with vanilla, sugar, crushed ice, and a pinch of salt. A doula named Jasmine Marsh makes breast-milk chai-latte cupcakes. She decorates them with areolas and nipples made of icing. A brisk online search yields recipes for lactation lasagna, breast-milk butter, breast-milk and mushroom risotto, mom's milk cheese, French toast with caramel sauce and breast milk, breast-milk yogurt, breast-milk smoothies, and momsicles. Momsicles are popsicles made of breast milk, apparently perfect for teething babies.

I have to assume that breast-milk recipes are something of a recent vogue, and that breast milk is not an ingredient women have used to cook and make soap with through the ages. But these days, thanks to pumps, many women have a large supply of breast milk on hand: much more than they need to feed their babies. And because breast milk is now widely perceived as something close to a magic elixir or, at the very least, a superfood, lots of people are eager to avail themselves of its celebrated health benefits. When an ice-cream store in London started selling breast-milk ice cream flavored with vanilla and lemon zest, at over twenty dollars a scoop, it sold out on the first day. Athletes have started using breast milk as an energy- and strength-building supplement. When a mother named Helen Fitzsimmons discovered her father had myeloma, she fed him expressed breast milk. They call it liquid gold, and demand is high.

Back in 1956, the founding mothers of La Leche League advocated breastfeeding as part of a broader platform that included mother-infant bonding, natural childbirth, the reaffirmation of maternal instincts, and stay-at-home mothering. Breastfeeding, they argued, was a crucial component of mother-infant bonding. The baby's primary need was for a close and nearly constant connection to its mother. Breastfeeding was beneficial because it enabled that physical intimacy.

La Leche and other breastfeeding advocates, like the Nursing Mothers of Greater Philadelphia, did not make the case that breast *milk* was beneficial to infants, or that it had any magical chemical properties. In part this may have been because, in 1956, little research had been done on the chemical composition of breast milk. Or they may have ignored such arguments as one more attempt to impose science on parenting. But the main reason they didn't make this case is that, along with many others, they believed that the benefits of breastfeeding came from mother-infant bonding.

Over time, the main arguments in favor of breastfeeding have shifted from the delivery system (the mother) to the product (human milk). Every breastfeeding campaign of the last twenty-five years has emphasized the "science" behind breastfeeding. The 2004 "Babies were born to be breastfed" campaign, sponsored by the US Department of Health and Human Services, was consciously designed to focus on science and risk. Each radio advertisement concluded with a male voice-over citing scientific research about the effects of breastfeeding: "Evidence shows that babies who are breastfed have 10 percent less risk of ear infection." By invoking the authority of science to highlight risk, some critics noted that the ads were consciously using scare tactics to induce mothers to breastfeed.

The 2012 Latch On NYC breastfeeding campaign in New York went one step further by omitting any reference to breastfeeding whatsoever. The campaign's slogan was "Breast milk is best for your baby." Another ad stated, "Nothing compares with breast milk." Still another distinguished between "mom-made" breast milk and "factory-made" formula, as if parents might be comparing different commodities, not different practices and commitments.

When I interviewed Dr. Thomas Farley, the architect of Latch On NYC, I asked him why the campaign focused on breast milk instead of breastfeeding. At first, Farley seemed surprised by my question. "We never thought of it that way," he responded, meaning they had not considered how feeding a baby breast milk from a bottle might differ from feeding a baby breast milk at the breast. "We were thinking of breast milk as opposed to formula, as alternative products." As I sat listening to him, I realized that Farley's description of breast milk as a *product* was the key to the whole public policy and marketing mindset. This apparently subtle shift from breastfeeding to breast milk had major implications—not only for mothers and babies, but also for business. That's when I began to wonder how this shift had happened. What, ultimately, was driving it?

AS I WOULD DISCOVER, the new focus on human milk is the result of many factors. Farley revealed the first one right away. When I asked him whether he thought feeding a baby expressed breast milk from a bottle was the same as feeding a baby from the breast, he paused for a long moment, then he started nodding slowly. "Yes, I can see what you're saying. I never thought about it that way. We never considered using the language of breast*feeding* is best for your baby." In retrospect, Farley could see that the Latch On NYC advertising campaign had sent the message that it was breast milk, not breastfeeding, that mattered most.

Later in our conversation, Farley seemed to indicate that the decision to focus on breast milk might have been something more than just an oversight. "I think we focused the advertising campaign on breast milk, not breastfeeding, because saying women should breast*feed* is just too big a change to the workplace, so you have to give them an easier alternative." The fact that most women in New York return to work soon after giving birth, combined with the structure of the workplace, made the health commissioner think it was unrealistic to promote breastfeeding. Because there is no maternity leave in the US, traditional breastfeeding is almost impossible for many women. Farley also pointed out that he was health commissioner under Michael Bloomberg, a mayor with strong business interests. Farley seemed to think that it was highly unlikely that Bloomberg would endorse any breastfeeding campaign that seemed, even by implication, to require maternity leave. Policy makers like Farley are sensitive to the need to get women back to work, and that sensitivity is one important reason for the shift from breastfeeding to breast milk.

But that's not the only reason. In medical journals and elsewhere, the term *breastfeeding* is starting to be replaced with *human lactation*. In case you're wondering, human lactation is the study of "the physiology and biochemistry of breast growth and development, milk synthesis, milk secretion, milk ejection, and the mechanics of breastfeeding." The irony here is that this term was popularized in part by breastfeeding advocates who were trying to gain professional status and legitimacy by redescribing themselves as "lactation consultants."

Although Surgeon General C. Everett Koop's 1984 workshop to promote breastfeeding produced very little in the way of practical results, it did identify "professional education" as one of six "core areas to be addressed for breastfeeding to become the community norm." In 1985, the International Board of Lactation Consultant Examiners (IBLCE) was constituted as an independent corporation to examine and certify professional lactation consultants. They developed an exam that combined "scientific facts and practical breastfeeding management principles." The International Lactation Consultants Association (ILCA) was formed in the same year. In 1993, the ILCA convened the first Lactation Education/Course Directors meeting to develop "international standards for professional lactation management education," and in 1999 the ILCA formalized a Professional Education Council. A board-certified lactation consultant gets to put the letters IBCLC (International Board Certified Lactation Consultant) after her name, and she is recognized as a medical professional by patients and peers, even if she does not have a medical or nursing degree.

Edith White, who was a breastfeeding educator and trainer before the term lactation consultant was ever invented, told me that her cohort of breastfeeding advocates had been very eager to professionalize their field. They felt it would offer them greater authority in dealing with clients and maybe even in dealing with nurses and doctors. In fact, many women who were already working as breastfeeding advocates, White included, received an honorary IBCLC designation without ever having to take the exam. The fact that most people who work in the field of breast-feeding support and advocacy are now certified lactation consultants, whose certification process includes the study of human lactation, is one of the factors that is gradually redefining breast-feeding to mean, simply, the production of human milk.

For the most part, however, lactation consultants have probably been unwitting accomplices in this major redefinition. Even if they don't follow all of La Leche League's principles, most lactation consultants probably share the League's belief that the defining feature of breastfeeding is that it offers an important opportunity for mother and infant bonding. Their role in redefining breastfeeding as the consumption of human milk has almost certainly been inadvertent.

But companies that manufacture breast pumps or use and sell human milk as a *product* are a different story. They have not only played an important role in this redefinition of breastfeeding; their efforts represent a well-developed corporate strategy.

The entire breast-pump industry depends on the premise that it's not *how* you feed your baby that matters but *what* you feed him or her. What babies need first and foremost, breast-pump manufacturers imply, is human milk. The Swiss company Medela once ran an ad that featured moms choosing among different brands of packaged breast milk in a supermarket.

Blurring the line between breastfeeding and human milk con-suption in this way has enabled these manufacturers to position themselves as breastfeeding advocates. Breast pumps are also effectively portrayed as products that *help* women breastfeed by maintaining a mother's milk supply when she is away from her baby. The fact that they do this by extracting breast milk with a machine, thereby eliminating the need for contact between mother and baby, is never mentioned.

Since 1961, Medela has focused exclusively on manufactur-ing breast pumps and related equipment such as bottles and storage containers. It has also funded extensive research on hu-man milk and human milk extraction. In the late 1990s, Medela started to fund the laboratory of Peter Hartmann, a biochemist at the University of Western Australia, to establish the Human Lactation Research Group, which studies "the mechanisms of removal of milk from the breast" to provide "an evidence base for the clinical management of human lactation." Medela iden-tifies the relationship between the company and the research group as a partnership.

Hartmann's background is actually in a field called rural sciences, and his main area of specialization and research is lactation in dairy cattle. His early research was funded by the Australian dairy industry. After completing his PhD, he held postdoctoral and research positions on lactation in dairy cat-tle in the UK, the United States, and Australia. As his bio on the Medela website adds, "Peter's research ranges from lactation in dairy animals and sows to lactation in women." One recent article is about piglets. Mostly, however, Hartmann now writes about human lactation, which is what Medela pays him for.

Medela's corporate interests and funding are in fact driving an entirely new branch of research that is rapidly transforming breastfeeding into "the clinical management of human lactation." In the decade between 2000 and 2009 alone, Hartmann wrote twenty-one research articles on breast milk and human lactation that were sponsored by Medela and published in some of the most important medical journals in the field, including *Pediatrics*, the *Journal of Human Lactation*, and *Breastfeeding Medicine*. These articles covered such topics as the composition of breast milk, the effect of vacuum profile on breast-milk expression (in other words, what vacuuming strength is ideal for expressing breast milk most efficiently), milk ejection using a pump, and how to standardize the fat content of human milk.

Medela has at least two very good reasons to fund this research. The first is to produce evidence that human milk is a valuable, even critical, commodity that has to be extracted from its source. The second is to inspire, develop, produce, and test new products. Medela describes Hartmann's research as directly responsible, for example, for Medela's "exclusive pumping pattern called 2-Phase Expression, which closely mimics a baby's natural nursing rhythm."

In fact, almost all of Medela's technological innovations seem geared toward making breastfeeding faster and more efficient. Medela boasts that "5 minutes with the Symphony Expression Phase can remove as much milk as an average 16 minute breastfeed." Medela's pump, in other words, is three times as efficient as your baby. Another paper by Hartmann and others apparently shows that "when used at Maximum Comfort Vacuum, 80% of expressed milk is removed in the first 7 minutes." According to Medela, Maximum Comfort Vacuum is "the highest vacuum a mother can tolerate and still be comfortable." Medela advises mothers to use Maximum Comfort Vacuum to maximize efficiency.

Increased speed and efficiency are, of course, highly desirable. They benefit employers by enabling mothers to pump breast milk at work in record time. And, obviously, they benefit mothers, some of whom are compelled to pump breast milk during a fifteen-minute break or even while driving. Still, it's hard to resist feeling that the whole idea of breastfeeding is being wildly distorted. Not long ago the primary goals of breastfeeding were the soft and fuzzy ones of nurture and comfort; now those goals have been replaced by the rhetoric of Taylorization, emphasizing efficiency and speed.

In 2006, Medela launched the Medela International Breastfeeding and Lactation Symposium, which takes place in different locations in Europe every April. In 2014 the symposium was held in Madrid. Over the course of the last decade, the symposium has gained increasing global visibility. The most recent meetings attracted between three hundred and four hundred medical professionals, lactation consultants, and representatives from the breast-pump manufacturing industry. They were there to hear presentations from nine or ten invited experts, most of whom are conducting research on the properties of human milk and human milk extraction. In 2013, Dr. Richard Schanler, the chair of the American Academy of Pediatrics (AAP) Section on Breastfeeding, and, as I mentioned earlier, the coauthor of the AAP Policy Statement on Breastfeeding and Human Milk, was the featured speaker. He presented his work on the medical benefits of human milk for premature infants.

As part of the American Academy of Pediatrics, the Section on Breastfeeding does not solicit independent funds. Members meet by telephone and communicate by e-mail, and the chair and other active board members perform their tasks on a purely voluntary basis, *pro bono*. They receive a small amount of funding from the AAP to hold occasional meetings. Schanler can only recall one instance when the Section on Breastfeeding received independent funding. It came from a breast-pump manufacturer, although Schanler did not mention which one. I asked Schanler if he perceived that funding, or his engagement as a featured speaker at the Medela conference, as a conflict of interest, and he said no, "because breast pump manufacturers are breastfeeding advocates."

Schanler's point here seems to have been that the interests of the AAP Section on Breastfeeding and Medela are aligned because they both advocate breastfeeding. But if breast-pump manufacturers are in fact advocates of human lactation, a practice that emphasizes the production and artificial extraction of human milk, is it really appropriate to call them *breastfeeding* advocates? The corporate interests of breast-pump manufacturers actually depend on mothers coming under increasing and sustained pressure to abandon breastfeeding in favor of breast pumping.

Many lactation consultants took note of that contradiction when Medela started to make, and market, bottles and nipples in 2008, which they claim violated the International Code of Marketing of Breastmilk Substitutes (the code originally designed to stop formula companies from marketing formula and feeding devices). The International Lactation Consultants Association, La Leche League International, the World Alliance for Breastfeeding Action, and the International Baby Food Action Network (IBFAN) have all cut ties with Medela: they do not accept Medela sponsorship, funding, or advertising.

Dr. Schanler, on the other hand, may come at this from a different perspective. The chair of the Section on Breastfeeding is actually, as I mentioned before, a neonatologist. His background in breastfeeding consists of "thirty or so years of research on human milk and feeding premature infants human milk." Premature infants almost never consume human milk by breastfeeding—they are usually too weak to coordinate breathing, sucking, and swallowing. They are often fed through a tube that goes into the stomach through their nose or mouth. Once they gain some strength, they may be fed by bottle. From Dr. Schanler's perspective, pumps and bottles are crucial to the success of "breastfeeding," and he told me he did not perceive any relevant distinction between breastfeeding and feeding a baby human milk from a bottle. His election to the chair of the Section on Breastfeeding, by the 500 members of the section, is another sign of the extent to which breastfeeding has been replaced by pumping and human milk consumption.

Dr. Schanler's background in feeding premature babies human milk also generated collaboration with a company called Prolacta Bioscience. Founded in 1999 and dedicated to "advancing the science of human milk," Prolacta uses human milk to manufacture nutritional supplements for premature babies. At its processing facility in City of Industry, California, just east of downtown Los Angeles, Prolacta uses human milk to make four different products designed for premature infants: a fortifier, a caloric fortifier, a premature infant formula, and standardized donor milk. In 2015, Prolacta had plans to process 3.4 million ounces—26,560 gallons—of milk. Its fortifiers cost $180 an ounce, and a premature baby is likely to use about $10,000 worth in a few weeks. Prolacta's products are used in roughly 150 of the 900 hospitals with neonatal intensive care units for extremely premature infants. According to Chief Executive Officer Scott Elster, the company is growing at the rate of 40 percent per year, although, since it is privately held, it does not disclose profits.

Almost everyone on Prolacta's board of directors has an extensive background in venture capital or the pharmaceutical industry. Ironically, one of them, Ernie Strapazon, retired from the Nestlé Corporation as president of the division that makes Good Start infant formulas. Prolacta has received $46 million in venture capital funds and, surprisingly to me at least, it is not the only company occupying this niche market.

Prolacta gets its raw material—human breast milk—through a network of affiliated milk donation sites across the country. For many years Prolacta solicited those donations for free. Given the projected increase in production, however, the company decided in 2014 to start paying women for the milk they provide the company. Still, at one dollar per ounce, Prolacta's rate is between one-half and one-third less than what a mother would make on the open market. Many breastfeeding advocates have expressed concern that Prolacta and other companies that use breast milk as a raw material are competing for breast milk with legitimate donor groups, like the Human Milk Banking Association of North America, a nonprofit organization that solicits milk donations for preterm infants in intensive care.

Like Medela, Prolacta Bioscience also has a corporate interest in promoting the idea that breast milk is a valuable resource. Since the mid-2000s, Prolacta has sponsored at least fifteen different studies concerning the chemical composition and benefits of human milk and the effects of the company's own products on preterm infants. In 2013 and 2014, two of the three clinical studies the company funded were conducted by Schanler and others, and Schanler coauthored two of the eight papers identified on the company's website as Prolacta Bioscience Published Papers. Those papers were all published in peer-reviewed medical journals, including the prestigious and highly influential *Journal of Pediatrics*, along with the disclosure that most of the authors "received financial support from Prolacta Bioscience." Although there are other doctors who appear to work more routinely with Prolacta, the company must have been pleased to have the chair of the AAP Section on Breastfeeding conducting clinical trials on the efficacy of its products and authoring its "published papers."

In fact it is not uncommon for doctors and scientists to conduct research that is funded by a company with a direct financial interest in the outcome of the research. Both Medela and Prolacta Bioscience have funded such research, and the results have been subsequently published in major peer-reviewed medical journals. It's hard to tell what proportion of medical research is funded by private interests. What *is* clear, however, is that corporations like Medela and Prolacta Bioscience are driving a research agenda that prioritizes human milk production and consumption over breastfeeding. Like formula before it, human lactation is big business.

PROLACTA BIOSCIENCE IS PART OF A much broader emerging market for human milk. Thanks to the practically universal use of breast pumps in the US, the freezers of American mothers are filling up, sometimes to the point of overflowing, with bags and bottles and ice cube trays of frozen breast milk. For the first time in the history of breastfeeding, there is actually a mismatch between supply and demand in the production of breast milk. And because this milk is widely believed to be liquid gold, women cannot bear to throw it away. Many mothers are proud of how much milk they produce. Friends of mine have often opened their freezers to show me their milk supply.

But eventually, once it becomes clear that their own precious babies will never be able to consume those giant freezers full of milk, mothers start to think of how to avoid letting it go to waste. And that's when they turn to the online market.

Like pumping itself, the market in breast milk is not unique to the United States, but it is much more common here than elsewhere. And, again, it appears to be largely driven by an over-supply of breast milk that has been driven by an overreliance on breast pumps—which has in turn been stimulated by effective corporate marketing campaigns and very significant govern-ment incentives. Women now dispatch their surplus supplies of milk across town, across the state, or across the country to strangers who want to feed their babies breast milk but cannot produce it themselves. Together, pumps and the Internet have revolutionized wet nursing.

Up until the early twentieth century, as we saw earlier, wet nursing was common. Working-class women used wet nurses so they could go out to work. Middle- and upper-class women used wet nurses as a matter of class privilege because it was un-fashionable or unseemly for a lady to breastfeed. Many other women used wet nurses if their baby was not thriving or their milk supply was inadequate.

But the key difference between old-fashioned wet nurs-ing and Internet-era wet nursing is that the earlier generation of women sold, and bought, a service. A wet nurse would take your baby—often for many months at a time—and nurse her. These days infant feeding is still being outsourced, but the focus is no longer on a service but a product: the sale and purchase of human milk, usually online.

This new development can be attributed in part to the long shadow cast by the Nestlé boycott. Popular outrage at the

multinational's cynical marketing practices in developing countries not only contributed to the rise in domestic breastfeeding
rates. It has also meant that a commitment to breastfeeding is
often paired with the demonization of formula. Formula feeding is so stigmatized that lots of American mothers who are
unable to produce breast milk now forgo formula, choosing
instead to buy unscreened, unpasteurized human milk online
from an unknown donor on an unregulated website. Literally
thousands of women are selling their milk online, and thousands more are buying it. In 2011, the *New York Times* reported
that "there were more than 13,000 postings on the four most
popular milk-sharing websites."

These milk-sharing websites are different from official milk
banks certified by the Human Milk Banking Association of
North America. Milk banks screen all donors to make sure they
are not carrying an infectious disease, and they pasteurize their
milk. But there are only twenty-two certified milk banks across
the United States and Canada—most states don't have any. And
almost all of the milk they collect is reserved for babies in neonatal intensive care units. The milk they sell costs between three
and six dollars per ounce. Mothers with healthy term babies are
not eligible to receive that milk, and many, presumably, could
not afford it.

On the other hand, parents can buy human breast milk at
www.onlythebreast.com for one to three dollars per ounce. This
website posts classified ads for both donors and buyers. The
New York Times describes the site as a Craigslist for breast milk.
Donors who advertise on the site tend to include information
about how healthy they are, how healthy their babies are, and
what they eat. Many claim they neither drink nor smoke. Some
say they are milk-bank certified. Some have a large supply of

frozen milk to sell; others offer to deliver pumped milk on a regular and ongoing basis.

Human milk is expensive. Between the ages of one and six months, babies eat roughly 25 ounces of milk per day. The normal range is between 19 and 30 ounces. If a family buys milk at the average cost of 2 dollars per ounce, they will pay 50 dollars per day, or 1,500 dollars per month, for breast milk. By contrast, formula costs about 100 dollars per month.

Human milk can also be dangerous. In 2013, the medical journal *Pediatrics* published research showing that breast milk purchased online was often infected. For the study, researchers anonymously purchased 101 samples of breast milk from online milk-sharing sites. They found that "most Internet samples (74%) would have failed HMBANA [Milk Banking Association of North America] criteria for feeding without pasteurization." "*Staphylococcus* sp were detected in a majority of Internet samples, and coliforms and *Streptococcus* sp were fairly common as well. Three Internet samples were contaminated with *Salmonella*." Follow-up research, published in March 2015, revealed that more than 10 percent of the samples were also diluted with more than 10 percent cow's milk.

These findings are worrisome, if hardly surprising. I personally would not expect that unscreened, unpasteurized milk bought online and shipped through the mail by an unknown donor would be reliably safe and free of infection or bacteria, or even reliably human milk.

Even more alarming is what those samples might have contained and, luckily, didn't. HIV can be transmitted through breast milk. So can tuberculosis, hepatitis A, hepatitis B, Lyme disease, syphilis, and chicken pox. Cytomegalovirus (CMV), a herpes virus, is fairly commonly transmitted through breast milk. And obviously milk bought online could contain alcohol, drugs, or medication.

Considering that even a small mistake, like leaving the milk unrefrigerated for too long, could make it unsafe, it is both un-believable and heartbreaking that so many parents suspend their disbelief to buy up whatever supplies they can. Breast milk is so highly regarded that the considerable risks that come with buying it through unregulated channels are routinely ignored or underestimated.

Some breastfeeding advocates oppose milk sharing precisely because of these risks and dangers. La Leche has long advised against wet nursing, cross nursing, and milk sharing through anything other than a formal milk bank. The AAP also recom-mends against buying human milk online and milk sharing.

Other breastfeeding activists and parents defend the prac-tice. They believe that consuming human milk is so import-ant that it's worth the risk. They insist, the evidence from the *Pediatrics* study notwithstanding, that the risk is small and, with shocking naïveté, that milk donors would never put another woman's baby at risk. This clubbish circling of the wagons can result in stunning leaps of logic. In an online response to the ev-idence that breast milk was often tainted, one breastfeeding ad-vocate argued that donors would have been aware that anyone buying only one ounce of milk was not using it for an infant, and therefore wouldn't have taken their usual safety precau-tions. What this bizarrely contorted argument suggests is that donors might maintain two separate milk stashes—of clean and infected milk—and that they reserve the infected milk for peo-ple they suspect of using it for fetishistic or other unsavory pur-poses. Although her example may not have been a good one, the thrust of her intervention was clear: anyone who breastfeeds is beyond reproach. A person who breastfeeds is necessarily a good person.

After the story about contaminated breast milk broke in 2013, www.eatsonfeets.org, another breast-milk-sharing website, stopped allowing people to post ads to buy and sell breast milk. Instead, the website now posts guidelines to promote safe breast-milk sharing and advocates a practice they call "community-based, commerce-free breast milk sharing." Their idea of community, however, is virtual, distributed across a potentially vast stretch of territory but connected online through the EatsOnFeets Facebook page. This is definitely not a home-spun cottage industry defined by face-to-face interactions or personal relationships. The term *commerce-free* refers to the organization's policy that milk "shared" through their online site must be donated, not sold. By eliminating the profit motive, they hope to attract only safe donors. But just in case, they also rely on an honor system that advises donors to "self-exclude" if they are unhealthy or using any dangerous substances, and they recommend donor screening.

Human Milk 4 Human Babies (HM4HB) is another organization that advocates and facilitates human milk sharing. This group uses "social media as a platform for local families to make real-life connections and come together as sustainable milk sharing communities." HM4HB allows people to post requests or offers of breast milk directly on its website. Often, mothers write that they need the milk immediately. On the HM4HB Connecticut Facebook webpage, someone asked: "Is there anyone in Enfield who can donate some milk today?" The women posting anonymously on this site propose meeting in parking lots and off highway exits. They explain that they post anonymously because someone—usually a mother or mother-in-law—disapproves of milk sharing. They don't want anyone to know what they're doing.

HM4HB seems to be the most radical of the organizations, less interested in the pragmatic logistics of making milk sharing safer, and more interested in retrieving not only breastfeeding, but communal and shared breastfeeding, as a political and feminist act. The group's mission statement directly challenges the warnings and recommendations of groups like La Leche and the AAP against unregulated breast-milk sharing. "Milk-sharing is a vital tradition that has been taken from us and it is crucial that we regain trust in ourselves, our neighbors, and in our fellow women." They want "milksharing and wet-nursing to be commonplace, and for babies to be fed at women's breasts whenever and wherever they need it." Their website states that they "stood their ground" when the Food and Drug Administration and Health Canada "issued warnings about the potential risks of milksharing."

CORPORATIONS THAT MANUFACTURE breast pumps and human milk by-products are not neutral and benevolent corporate funders. They are pushing a research agenda that has transformed breastfeeding—and yet remains largely unacknowledged. As a result, the consequences of this transformation are rarely considered. We have no idea if feeding a baby breast milk offers the same benefits as breastfeeding. There is no research that distinguishes between the benefits associated with breastfeeding as defined by the practice of feeding an infant at the breast and benefits associated with feeding a baby human milk from a bottle. Since the latter is gradually replacing the former and is generally treated as a fully equivalent alternative, this research gap is significant. And so is the silence around it.

The bottom line is that nobody knows for sure whether bottle-feeding human milk offers the same benefits as mother-to-infant breastfeeding. Nonetheless, the pediatricians and breastfeeding researchers I spoke to tend to believe they are not the same thing. Dr. Farley, for example, believes the actual *health* benefits of breastfeeding are limited to small differences in susceptibility to infections. From the perspective of health alone, he says, the benefits are pretty small. He believes that the real value of breastfeeding is related to its psychosocial effects. By psychosocial he means long-term psychological effects that would improve the well-being of our society. "It's hard for me to really say how big a public health issue it is because, you know, in the short run, what breastfeeding does is it prevents against infections, and it may have other benefits that seem pretty small. But if in fact it has psychosocial effects, then that could have all kinds of down-stream benefits way beyond just preventing infections. It could change, for instance, substance abuse and anti-social behavior. I have no evidence for that, but even without hard data, I do tend to believe as a pediatrician that there is a psychosocial benefit there."

Those potential benefits, he believes, would not come from the chemical properties of human milk; they would come from the mother-infant bonding that goes along with feeding a baby at the breast. Farley did not shy away from taking the logical next step: "Of course if the benefit is psychosocial, then that would mean that pumping is not as good. Yes, that's gotta be right." This puts Farley in the same camp as old-style breast-feeding advocates and attachment parents.

Even doctors who are not necessarily focused on the potential psychosocial benefits of maternal-infant bonding believe that some of the most important benefits associated with breastfeeding come from intense interaction between mother and infant and not from the consumption of human milk alone. If breastfeeding does indeed have any positive effect on cognitive development, for example, there are reasons to think that human milk alone would not have that same effect.

We saw earlier that one of the most striking findings from Kramer's PROBIT study was that breastfeeding did seem to have some positive effect on cognitive development. It turns out that this finding is at odds with some other research on cognitive development. Most significantly, it is at odds with the 2009 AHRQ meta-analysis that evaluated all the most recent studies on this particular issue. That report found "little or no evidence for an association between breastfeeding and cognitive performance in children."

Why then is the PROBIT study a relative outlier on this particular issue? It could be because almost none of the breastfeeding women who participated in the Belarus study used a pump. Kramer estimates that about "five women out of the seventeen thousand women enrolled in the study" might have used a pump. In other words, almost every single one of the breastfeeding women in the study fed her infant at the breast. If it's breastfeeding *at the breast* that matters, US studies would be less likely to find any cognitive benefit because American studies count both babies who drink human milk from a bottle and babies who feed at the breast as breastfeeding.

The possibility that the PROBIT cognitive development findings were driven by the fact that the breastfeeding Belarusian women all fed their babies at the breast is a plausible theory. And there are two other good reasons to think breastfeeding is more important for cognitive development than human milk. Many researchers have suggested that breastfeeding affects

neurocognitive outcomes because of the intense interaction between mothers and babies who breastfeed. They speculate that,
in general, women who breastfeed engage more intimately and
consistently with their children. They talk to them while they
are breastfeeding and look down at them, making eye contact
and smiling. Kramer thinks that the quality of this intimate interaction might explain why the biggest difference they found
was in verbal IQ. He also likes to cite a famous study in which
rat babies that were licked and groomed by their mothers were
better at running mazes and remembering cues than rats that
were removed from their mothers.

There is also a third potential reason Kramer finds compelling: there is nothing in breast milk that could reasonably be
expected to affect intelligence. Kramer explained the chemical factors at play. "I would think breastfeeding [as opposed
to human milk] would be most likely to make a difference on
the neurocognitive outcomes because we can see what some
of these molecules—oligosaccharides, IGA, lactoferrin—we
can see in vitro and in animal models how they work to reduce
gastrointestinal and respiratory infections. Those mechanisms
are pretty well worked out. So we know enough about what's in
breast milk to know that it's probably insufficient to explain the
effect [on cognitive outcomes]."

A 2011 article in the *American Journal of Public Health* suggests that expressed milk may also be less effective in preventing
infection than breast milk that comes directly from the breast,
or could in fact *cause* infection. Expressed milk is often refrig-
erated or frozen. Refrigeration and freezing can cause both degradation of milk components and the growth of bacteria. Milk
expressed with a pump also makes contact with nipple shields
and valves, bottles, and teats. Each one of these parts could be

contaminated. Apparently some research has shown that "bacterial counts are higher in milk expressed with a pump than in milk expressed by hand."

The National Immunization Survey, which is the source for data on breastfeeding initiation and duration, does not distinguish between breastfeeding and pumping. As a result we don't really know how much milk breastfeeding babies are getting from bottles and how much they are getting from the breast. "At a minimum," says the *American Journal of Public Health* article, "feeding at the breast should be distinguished from feeding expressed milk, and the durations of each practice should be ascertained."

Kramer also believes that the differences between feeding a baby at the breast and feeding a baby human milk should be the subject of a specific research agenda. Toward the end of our conversation about the PROBIT study, he expressed surprise about the fact that such studies have not yet started. "In a country where that's very common, where pumping is common, they *should* be doing that research." When he presents the PROBIT findings on breastfeeding and cognitive development, Kramer routinely admits that scientists don't know whether it's something in the milk or maternal-infant interaction that makes the difference. And he emphasizes "that really needs to be studied."

Kramer concedes that this kind of research is complicated and probably expensive, but he also says that it is hardly impossible. He thinks that maybe science hasn't caught up with the changing norms of breastfeeding. Maybe it's just inertia, or maybe nobody has thought of it yet.

But it's also possible that there is not a great deal of enthusiasm, at least in some quarters. Through the National Institutes of Health, the US government funds $30.3 billion dollars of medical research annually in the United States. If new research began to reveal that feeding a baby human milk from a bottle did not confer even the limited or "modest" positive effects associated with traditional breastfeeding, that evidence would directly contradict every major breastfeeding advocacy initiative since 2009. It would also generate a powerful argument for six months of federally mandated maternity leave, or changing the structure of the workplace in a way that gave mothers regular access to their breastfeeding babies, or both.

Breast-pump manufacturers, and more recently the companies that make human milk–based products, have also been a leading funder of breastfeeding research. They have been partly responsible for shifting research away from breastfeeding and toward the chemical composition of human milk and its efficient extraction. It seems unlikely that such companies as Medela, Ameda, or Prolacta Bioscience would be eager to fund research that might directly undercut their financial interests. Those interests are directly tied to the claim that the benefits of breastfeeding come from human milk, regardless of how it is delivered.

It's perfectly clear why certain constituencies have an interest in promoting the idea that human milk is a valuable commodity. Those constituencies include the companies that produce the pumps that extract the resource, the companies and artisanal chefs who use human milk as a raw material in their production process, and even exclusive pumpers and some of those moms who are making a tidy profit selling their milk online.

We are still in the earliest stages of the transition from breastfeeding to the consumption of human milk, and the implications of that transition are not yet clear. With the provision of free breast pumps to every mother in America, however, human milk consumption may soon come close to replacing breastfeeding altogether. As production increases, and the market grows more highly regulated, mothers of means may start to reason, as some already have, that they can more easily buy breast milk on the open market than produce it themselves. Other mothers will realize that they can make money by engaging in a highly personalized form of commodity extraction. Once breastfeeding breaks down into the production and consumption of human milk, it will create the usual divisions and conflicts of interests that characterize the relationship between producers and consumers in every market. It's worth thinking about what the ethical and legal implications of those exchanges will be, because the train has long since left the station.

CHAPTER 7

"Mother's Milk Can Kill Babies!"
Lactivism and HIV

In 1981, the Centers for Disease Control and Prevention (CDC) first reported five cases of a rare lung infection among gay men with compromised immune systems in Los Angeles. By the end of 1981, five to six new cases of the mysterious disease were being reported each week, and by the time the CDC first referred to it as acquired immune deficiency syndrome (AIDS), in July 1982, one to two new cases were being reported every day in the United States.

The emerging AIDS crisis seemed far removed from the Nestlé boycott and the concerns of breastfeeding advocates, who, at that point, in the early 1980s, had reason to celebrate. In 1981, the same year AIDS was first identified in the US, the World Health Assembly adopted the International Code of Marketing of Breast-milk Substitutes, limiting formula marketing strategies. By 1984, even Nestlé had agreed to abide by the code, and the world's leading public health organizations had joined the fight to reestablish breastfeeding as the best practice for infant feeding in developing countries. The soaring rates of infant mortality that accompanied the rise of formula use in poor countries had given breastfeeding a new moral authority. In the US too, breastfeeding had taken on new life. Between 1971 and 1984, breastfeeding initiation rates jumped dramatically, from 24 to 60 percent.

Not only did AIDS and breastfeeding seem to have absolutely nothing to do with one another, their prospects as health issues seemed radically different as well. Between the heightened commitment to breastfeeding advocacy around the world and the restrictions the new marketing code imposed on formula companies, it seemed that the devastating health crisis caused in many parts of the global south by widespread formula use was finally being addressed. The AIDs crisis, on the other hand, was just beginning to make its presence felt, not only among medical professionals but among the general public—and there was no end in sight.

But in December 1982, these two apparently distinct issues converged. That month CDC reported four cases of babies in the United States who had died of unexplained cellular immunodeficiency and opportunistic infections. Two of the babies' mothers were intravenous drug users. One of the mothers had died of pneumonia. The health status of the other two sets of parents was unknown. None of the babies had received blood transfusions or blood products prior to illness. The CDC was also investigating six other cases of babies who had died with apparently similar immune profiles and twelve more children who were alive but suffering from various AIDS-associated conditions including failure to thrive, candidiasis, and resistant pneumonia. The CDC speculated that these cases might mean that AIDS was being transmitted from mother to child, either in utero or shortly after birth. Two years later, in April 1985, the highly regarded British medical journal, *The Lancet,* published the first evidence that HIV could be transmitted through breastfeeding.

EXPERTS NOW BELIEVE THAT THE FIRST AIDS epidemic occurred in Kinshasa, Zaire (now Democratic Republic of the Congo), in the 1970s, when a large number of people died of opportunistic infections, including tuberculosis, Kaposi's sarcoma, and pneumonia. But it was not until the 1980s that the disease began its devastating sweep through Central and East Africa. As early as 1983, researchers confirmed twenty-six cases of AIDS in Kigali, Rwanda, and thirty-eight in Kinshasa, Zaire. By 1985 those numbers had grown exponentially: 35 percent of Ugandan truck drivers who were tested and 30 percent of the Ugandan army were found to be HIV positive. In neighboring Kenya, President Daniel arap Moi declared AIDS a national disaster that threatened the country's very existence.

In 1985, two thousand activists, public health officials, and doctors from all over the world attended the world's first international conference on AIDS in Atlanta, and the World Health Organization (WHO) soon followed up with a second meeting to initiate "concerted worldwide action against the AIDS epidemic." The director of WHO estimated that "as many as 10 million people worldwide could already be infected with HIV," and experts projected that those numbers would multiply "epidemically." Even in the United States, where the disease was still concentrated among gay men, experts projected that 2 to 3 million Americans would be infected with HIV by 1995. Nobody doubted that, especially in Sub-Saharan Africa and South Asia, millions of people would be infected and die of HIV/AIDS before the end of the decade.

It had also become clear that HIV/AIDS would eventually have its greatest impact among women and young people. Although HIV first manifested in the United States as a disease more or less confined to gay men, in Africa and most of the rest of the developing world HIV/AIDS is often transmitted through heterosexual contact. As a result, the main at-risk groups have been women who have multiple sexual partners and women who have sex with men who have multiple sexual partners. In 1986, 85 percent of sex workers in Nairobi were infected with HIV. Globally, women account for more than half of people infected with HIV, and in Africa women account for almost 60 percent. Among young people aged fifteen to twenty-four, a ten-year range that accounts for almost one-third of the total infections worldwide, girls outnumber boys two to one.

Because AIDS is transmitted primarily through sexual contact, it is especially prevalent among women of reproductive age. In fact, HIV/AIDS is the leading cause of death worldwide among women ranging in age from roughly fifteen to forty. In the countries of East and Southern Africa, which were hardest hit by the epidemic, WHO estimated that, in 1989, roughly 30 percent of pregnant women were infected with HIV.

The very large number of pregnant women infected with HIV has had tragic consequences for infants and children. AIDS is most commonly transmitted through sexual intercourse and needle sharing. But the third-most common mode of transmission is mother-to-child transmission around birth. As early as 1985, the *New York Times* reported that, in Africa, one in five people infected with HIV was a child.

WHO and UNICEF estimated that six hundred thousand babies were newly infected with HIV every year during the

1990s. Between 1994 and 1997, the number of children who were living with HIV/AIDS tripled. In its 1998 Progress of Nations Report, UNICEF estimated that "by the year 2005, 48% of all child deaths under the age of five will be because of AIDS." In 2000, experts projected that the under-five mortality rate in the worst hit areas would increase by over 100 percent by 2010. In the twenty-five years since 1990, more than half a million babies have been newly infected with HIV each year.

Nine out of ten children infected with HIV are infected through their mother—either during pregnancy, labor and delivery, or breastfeeding. The fetus may contract HIV in utero, or through exposure to the mother's blood during delivery, especially if the mother's water breaks more than four hours before delivery, if she has a vaginal delivery, or if there is trauma or bleeding at birth.

The crucial 1985 article that linked breastfeeding with HIV transmission was confirmed by follow-up research throughout the second half of the 1980s. Not only had medical testing shown that HIV was present in breast milk, but scientific research, including prospective studies among infants born to HIV-infected mothers, confirmed that breastfed babies were more likely to be infected than formula-fed babies. Research also showed that duration mattered—the longer a baby breastfed, the more likely she was to be infected with HIV.

After 1989, this research became even more robust with the development of a more sophisticated method of HIV testing. Up until 1989, researchers could only assess the transmission of HIV through breastfeeding among the small cohort of babies who had not been exposed to HIV in utero or at birth. Because the test actually measured the existence of HIV antibodies, and babies may retain some of their mother's antibodies for up to eighteen months after birth, babies born to HIV-infected mothers sometimes tested positive for HIV antibodies even if they were HIV negative. So, even though there was evidence that HIV was being transmitted through breastfeeding, there was no way of measuring the relative risk of transmission in utero, at birth, or through breastfeeding.

In 1989, however, scientists developed a new method of HIV testing (PCR, polymerase chain reaction) that detects the genetic material of HIV rather than HIV antibodies. This new test made it easier to establish whether babies were infected before or during birth or through breastfeeding. In 1992, *The Lancet* published the definitive meta-analysis of the existing research on this subject, revealing that the risk of HIV transmission through breastfeeding was between 14 and 29 percent. In absolute numbers, roughly 220,000 babies around the world were infected with HIV each year through breastfeeding alone.

Following the 1985 discovery that breastfeeding could transmit HIV, the CDC and the American Academy of Pediatrics (AAP) immediately issued a recommendation that women infected with HIV should avoid breastfeeding. Officials in Europe, Canada, Australia, and New Zealand followed suit. But breastfeeding activists in those countries pointedly ignored that advice.

Edith White was one of them. She still remembers the skepticism that the CDC's recommendation provoked in the lactivist community. "The politically correct reaction on the part of us breastfeeding advocates," White told me, "was 'oh there are more of these white men doctors we've all had bad advice from!'" She and her colleagues at Nursing Mothers dismissed the CDC recommendations because they came from a medical establishment they not only distrusted, but against which they had joined forces in the first place. Lactivists like White suspected that the CDC was probably pandering to the formula companies, and some of them were angry at the very suggestion that women's bodies could be lethal to their babies. Many of them refused to believe that breast milk could transmit HIV, and others worried that, even if it did, publicizing that information would undermine their breastfeeding campaigns.

By the early 1990s, the lactation consultancy business that White and her partner had started in 1976 was flourishing, and breastfeeding rates in the US were growing steadily. But like the vast majority of breastfeeding advocates in the US, White remained silent about the potential danger of HIV transmission through breastfeeding. She told me that the training courses they offered WIC counselors always included a review of medical research. "Say we went to Milwaukee every May, and then every year we would provide an update on what's been published in the medical journals, to keep them abreast of the research. And at that point of course the research was all very positive." Eventually though, White explained, it was impossible to ignore the fact that the evidence was changing. "All of a sudden you couldn't help but notice that if you did a search for breastfeeding at the Harvard Medical Library, you would come up with a lot of HIV articles! Oh my God! By the early 1990s, I started to think we should pass this information along in our training."

White realized this information could be particularly relevant to the WIC counselors they were training. "Some of those offices were in places where their clients were very likely to be potentially exposed to HIV." But even though some WIC clients had partners who were injecting drugs, or had multiple partners, White noticed that the WIC counselors she worked with were reluctant to address these issues. "WIC counselors were comfortable primarily talking about nutrition. They were happy to recommend a good source of vitamin C. But to talk about women's intimate partners or sex lives?" White answered her own question by mimicking the reaction of a WIC counselor: "Well, I just wouldn't be *comfortable!*"

In fact, even though many people realized that "*obviously* breast milk is a body fluid that transfers HIV," nobody in White's cohort thought it wise to publicize that information. White describes eventually coming to terms with the news in a voice that, even today, is tinged with horror and sorrow. "You can't help but accept the very sad news. Mother's milk can kill babies! There's no doubt about it. It was awful." For many committed lactivists, then and now, breast milk is by definition good and wholesome. The idea that it might harm or even kill babies is often literally unthinkable.

Ultimately, White's business disbanded over the question of whether to include information about HIV in breastfeeding advocacy training sessions. To this day, WIC has never really directly addressed the issue of HIV and breastfeeding. It didn't develop an official policy for dealing with clients who were HIV positive until 1999—fourteen years after the publication of *The Lancet* article revealing that breastfeeding could transmit HIV. And as recently as 2014, the unofficial policy was still "don't ask, don't tell." In a phone conversation, the director of WIC for Western New York told me that counselors don't ask about the HIV status of their clients because it would be an invasion of privacy. But because they do not mention HIV at all, counselors are left in the tricky position of recommending breastfeeding to all their clients and hoping that those who are HIV positive will find out on their own about the risk that breastfeeding poses to their babies.

BY THE MID-1990S, WHITE HAD GROWN into an important figure in the world of breastfeeding advocacy, a world she had been deeply involved in for over twenty years. Her book *The Breastfeeding Handbook* was published in 1980, and a revised edition written in collaboration with a second author appeared in 1989. Her numerous pamphlets on breastfeeding were sold to doctors and public health agencies all over the country. She was invited to the Surgeon General's Workshop on Breastfeeding and Human Lactation in 1984.

And in 1996, UNICEF invited White to be one of two American delegates to an international breastfeeding colloquium in Bangkok, Thailand. It was the first breastfeeding training conference ever held, and it was cosponsored by UNICEF, WHO, and the World Alliance for Breastfeeding Action. What White learned at that conference changed her life.

By 1996, eleven years had passed since the first reports of HIV transmission through breast milk. It had been four years since the publication of research showing that 14 to 29 percent of breastfed babies who were born to HIV-positive mothers would contract HIV. In some parts of the developing world, up to 30 percent of pregnant women were infected with HIV. But here, at this breastfeeding colloquium convened by the most important health policy organizations in the world, it was as if HIV didn't exist. Already concerned that breastfeeding advocates in the United States were ignoring the fact that HIV could be transmitted through breast milk, White was shocked to discover that the problem was even worse among international health organizations. Although public health officials in North America, Europe, Australia, and New Zealand had responded quickly to reports that HIV could be transmitted through breastfeeding, changing their infant-feeding recommendations for women infected with HIV, international organizations like WHO and UNICEF did nothing. It was after that conference that White began the long and painful process of discovery that would ultimately lead to her 1999 book, *Breastfeeding and HIV/AIDS: The Research, the Politics, the Women's Responses.*

In developing countries, international public health organizations had been advocating breastfeeding for over a decade. The 1981 International Code of Marketing had been celebrated as a landmark victory. Nestlé had finally agreed to implement the code in 1984, and in 1985 global support for breastfeeding was at an all-time high. For many world health officials and health-care workers in the developing world, breastfeeding was one of the main weapons against infant mortality. Protests against Nestlé had persuaded them that breastfeeding could dramatically reduce the number of deaths from malnutrition and diarrhea—the number-one cause of infant death in the developing world. Like their lactivist counterparts in the United States, these world health officials were concerned that publicizing the link between breastfeeding and HIV would undermine their breastfeeding advocacy campaigns. Defending breastfeeding was more important than defending babies' lives. And so in 1987 WHO issued the recommendation that mothers should continue to breastfeed "irrespective of their HIV infection status." In its 1987 Global AIDS Plan, WHO stated that "the probability of HIV transmission through breastfeeding was apparently small."

World health organizations continued to downplay the risk of transmitting HIV via breastfeeding throughout the 1980s. In its 1989 report *State of the World's Children*, UNICEF reported that "breastfeeding is not a significant means of transmitting

AIDS," despite growing evidence to the contrary. They insisted that the risk of contracting HIV through breastfeeding was low and that the relative risk of dying of diarrhea or malnutrition caused by formula feeding was much higher. On the basis of these two misguided premises, they continued to recommend breastfeeding as the lesser of two evils. As Dr. Francis Miro, the beleaguered chief of obstetrics and gynecology at Makerere University Medical Hospital in Kampala, Uganda, told a *New York Times* reporter, "Twenty-seven percent of babies born to infected mothers become infected from breastfeeding. In rural areas 85% of babies will die from dirty water used in formula." His account of the statistics must have reflected his feeling of being caught in a catch-22, but, if he was accurately quoted by the *New York Times*, his numbers were way off.

World health organizations in fact routinely pitted the risk of HIV transmission against the risk of formula feeding in a way that made the former seem almost trivial by comparison. But such comparisons were misleading. In fact, the risk of infant mortality from malnutrition or diarrhea varies widely, but there is no place in the world, including rural Uganda, where 85 percent of babies die, let alone die from formula feeding alone.

In fact, the infant mortality rate in Uganda was 8.6 percent in 1988. In Afghanistan, which has the highest infant mortality rate in the world, it was 15 percent. In Botswana, by contrast, the infant mortality rate in 1985 was forty-seven deaths per thousand live births, or 4.7 percent; of those, about 25 percent of deaths could be attributed to malnutrition and diarrhea. This means that just over 1 percent of babies in Botswana could plausibly be said to be dying of malnutrition and diarrhea. Clearly that represents a devastating number of infant deaths.

But, thankfully, it is a far cry from the 85 percent that may have been cited by Miro.

Finally, after the publication of the 1992 meta-analysis revealing that 14 to 29 percent of breastfed babies born to HIV-infected mothers were infected with HIV, scientists started to conduct research explicitly measuring the relative risk of HIV transmission through breastfeeding compared with death through formula feeding. Those studies uniformly concluded that there were very few places in the developing world where the risk of dying of malnutrition or diarrhea was higher than the risk of contracting HIV (and dying) through breastfeeding. The weight of the evidence strongly suggested that the risk of mortality from HIV almost always exceeded the risks associated with infant formula.

And yet even after 1992, by which time the extent of the risk of HIV transmission from breastfeeding was clear, WHO and UNICEF failed to change course. As White demonstrated starkly in her book, both organizations effectively ignored the unfolding tragedy of AIDS-related infant deaths and continued to recommend that women should breastfeed their babies regardless of their HIV status.

The failure of world health organizations to discuss the relationship between breastfeeding and HIV in their publications during this time suggests more than oversight: it seems deliberate. In 1993, UNICEF's *State of the World's Children* report made no mention of HIV/AIDS even though, in that year alone, six hundred thousand children were newly infected with HIV. UNICEF also published a report called *AIDS: The Second Decade*, which devoted only one sentence to children—even though UNICEF is an organization dedicated to the protection of children—and failed to offer any explanation for how children contract HIV. In 1993, WHO published a book called

Breastfeeding: The Technical Basis and Recommendations for Action. That book discussed the transmission of HIV through breastfeeding under the heading "spreading false rumors."

Over the course of the next two years, a growing body of research confirmed the worst: that AIDS was becoming the leading cause of death for children under five in many parts of the developing world and that breastfeeding was a major means of HIV transmission. One 1995 study reported that "nine out of nine Saudi Arabian babies breastfed by HIV positive mothers became infected." Similar studies reported rates of 48 percent infection in India and 35 percent infection in Malawi, among babies breastfed by mothers with HIV.

And yet UNICEF's 1996 *State of the World's Children* report mentioned AIDS only in passing, to say that many children had been orphaned by the AIDS epidemic. The report also lamented the fact that the mortality rate for children under the age of five was going up in Sub-Saharan Africa and South Asia, without explaining why. Similarly, in 1997, WHO issued a fact sheet called "Reducing Mortality from Major Childhood Killer Diseases" that failed to mention HIV/AIDS, even though AIDS had become the leading cause of death for children in most countries in East and Southern Africa. Although AIDS was the leading cause of pediatric death in Zambia, for example, the section about major childhood killers in Zambia made no mention of AIDS at all.

At the time, many scientists and nutritionists accused UNICEF and WHO of ignoring facts "in their zeal to promote breastfeeding." In a 1998 interview with a *New York Times* reporter, Dr. Susan Holck, an expert on breastfeeding at WHO, said she was "struck by how much denial there was around 1990 of the evidence we had that HIV could be transmitted through breastfeeding." That denial, she explained, "was undoubtedly fed by people who had invested so much in promoting breastfeeding and feared what confirmation of that transmission might do to the gains that were made in breastfeeding." Dr. Miriam Labbok, the director of the World Health Organization Collaborating Center on Breastfeeding from 1992 to 1996, may have been one of those people. Labbok has often publicly expressed the concern that the AIDS pandemic poses a grave danger to breastfeeding advocacy.

Many health officials in developing countries were also furious about the willful blindness of the world health organizations. A Zimbabwean delegate to the Bangkok colloquium White attended told her privately that there were hand-lettered signs posted all over the capital of Harare that said "UNICEF Kills Babies," referring to the organization's insistence that mothers infected with HIV should breastfeed. In a spectacular understatement, Zambian gynecologist Mavis Sianga complained that "it is rather unfair that women in developing countries must risk passing on the infection just because WHO and UNICEF want to keep their programs flying."

African delegates to the 1997 World Health Assembly also criticized WHO and UNICEF for failing to disseminate information about the transmission of HIV through breastfeeding. Their statement included the following pointed question: "Are we to accept that our children's survival should be compromised by the risk of infant AIDS in the cruelest sense through the promotion of unlimited, unmodified, and unchallenged breastfeeding policies?" In particular, health officials in Africa were furious about this apparent double standard in advice: "In the affluent industrialized countries WHO advises HIV-infected women to stop breastfeeding, while in developing countries HIV-infected women are advised to carry on breastfeeding."

It was not until 1998 that world health organizations revised their infant-feeding guidelines for mothers infected with HIV. In its major 1998 report on HIV transmission through breast-feeding, UNAIDS, a consortium drawn from UNICEF, United Nations Development Programme, United Nations Popula-tion Fund, United Nations Educational, Scientific and Cultural Organization, WHO, and the World Bank, finally stated that "for an HIV-infected woman to eliminate completely the risk of HIV transmission through breastfeeding, she needs to feed her infant from birth with suitable replacements for breast milk (such as commercial infant formula or home-prepared formula made from modified animal milks)." International health orga-nizations finally acknowledged that breastfeeding accounted for "up to 40 percent" of all cases of infant HIV infection and rec-ommended that mothers infected with HIV feed their babies formula.

Since then, progress in the medical treatment of HIV has reduced the risk of mother-to-infant transmission. Now that more mothers and babies have access to antiretroviral medica-tions that reduce their viral load, most publications identify the risk as 5 to 20 percent. Nevertheless, according to a WHO re-port published in 2008, approximately 420,000 infants are still infected with HIV each year, and between one third and one half of those infections—between 140,000 and 210,000—could be attributed to breastfeeding alone. What these numbers mean is that in the thirty-five or so years since the epidemic began, between 4.9 million and 7.35 million babies have been infected with HIV through breastfeeding alone.

WHEN WHO AND UNICEF ISSUED recommendations that HIV positive mothers should feed their babies formula in 1998 and began to distribute free formula in poor countries, lactivists were dismayed. This was precisely what they had been trying to prevent for thirteen years. La Leche League issued a statement in June of that year suggesting there was not enough evidence to support the WHO decision. "Some researchers have isolated HIV in human milk.... Yet other studies have not shown there to be a very high risk of transmission through breastfeeding." The statement also claimed that many studies had not differentiated between viral fragments of HIV and intact HIV virus within the cells in milk; only the latter type could replicate and therefore be considered infectious.

A few months later, the February/March 1999 issue of La Leche's magazine *Leaven* warned that "for the 93 percent of infants worldwide who are *not* HIV positive, there is a danger that public information about the risks of transmission of HIV in breast milk could cause an overall reduction in breastfeeding." They concluded that "fear of HIV transmission is the biggest threat to breastfeeding in the Third World, where a large fraction of women are HIV-positive."

Many of the advocates who feared for the future of breastfeeding programs simply rejected the evidence showing that breastfeeding could cause harm. They refused to relinquish the dream of "mother's milk" as the perfect solution. Some of them no doubt calculated that such an admission would be a strategic mistake—the thin edge of the wedge that would ultimately undermine breastfeeding altogether. Others were so deeply committed to the belief that breastfeeding was right and good, they simply could not countenance any other possibility. Like White and her colleagues, many international breastfeeding advocates were already suspicious of the medical establishment, which had recommended formula feeding to new mothers during the 1950s and 1960s, and were predisposed to doubt scientific evidence.

For some of these hard-core lactivists, AIDS denialism offered a lifeline. Led by the widely discredited UC Berkeley scientist Peter Duesberg, AIDS denialists are a small group of journalists and pseudoscientists who disseminate the idea that HIV either does not exist or that it does not cause AIDS. Most notoriously, AIDS denialism gained international prominence when it was publicly embraced by former South African president Thabo Mbeki.

For more than thirty years, the thousands of scientists who conduct research on HIV/AIDS have built an indisputable body of evidence about the HIV retrovirus and how it converts from HIV to AIDS. Although denialists claim to be advancing an alternative scientific theory, they are almost universally perceived as quacks. But they have found a ready audience among lactivists, because their insistence that AIDS does not exist extends readily to the claim that HIV is either not present in breast milk or not transmitted through breastfeeding.

In 2001, La Leche League International invited another infamous AIDS denialist, David Crowe, to speak at its international conference in Chicago. David Crowe is a Canadian journalist whose scientific credentials are limited to an undergraduate degree in biology and mathematics from Lakehead University in Ontario. Crowe is nevertheless the founder and president of the Alberta Reappraising AIDS Society and the president of Rethinking AIDS. He is closely allied with Duesberg, who is on the board of directors of Rethinking AIDS. Both the Alberta Reappraising AIDS Society and Rethinking AIDS publish the work of so-called dissident scientists, provide a wide range of questionable medical information to AIDS patients, and solicit donations. Crowe also provides medical advice online to people who have stopped taking their HIV/AIDS medications. A visit to the Reappraising AIDS website in 2014 revealed that Crowe had turned his attention to Ebola, which he called "another mythical virus." When I asked him about it, Crowe explained that nobody had ever "purified a virus, let alone proved that it was the cause of the disease." He also had some more tangential reasons for believing that Ebola is not a virus.

At the 2001 La Leche League International Conference in Chicago, however, Crowe was still focused on HIV, and he delivered a presentation called "Infectious HIV in Breast Milk: Fact or Fantasy?" His claim was that antigen tests cannot be used to prove the existence of HIV in breast milk; that the HIV virus has never been isolated; and that no HIV test had ever been properly "validated." He also alleged that the PCR test (used to more accurately pinpoint whether babies were infected in utero or after birth through breastfeeding) was, on the one hand, so sensitive that it detected levels of HIV that were too small to cause disease but on the other hand unable to detect the presence of "infectious HIV."

He concluded by offering breastfeeding activists a "challenge." They could "accept current dogmas about HIV, breastfeeding and AIDS, and watch breastfeeding retreat in the Third World" or they could "ignore majority opinions. Weigh the Evidence. Be prepared to Paddle up the Creek, Build a Summer Igloo, Sail into the Wind!" Crowe was invited to the conference by Marian Tompson, who also chaired his panel and introduced him.

Tompson is one of the original seven founding mothers of La Leche League. She was also the president of the organization for twenty-four years, from 1956 to 1980. She has been a member of the Advisory Council of the World Alliance for Breastfeeding Action since 1996. She is still on the fourteen-member

Advisory Board of La Leche League International, and she is a La Leche League International Accredited Leader. She often represents La Leche League at local, national, and international conferences. There she often sits on panels with AIDS denialists and expresses the view that there is no conclusive proof that HIV is transmitted through breastfeeding.

Tompson took up Crowe's challenge by forming an organization called AnotherLook, which challenges the medical community's approach to breastfeeding and HIV/AIDS. AnotherLook is a nonprofit organization that disseminates the "research" and position papers of AIDS denialists. Like La Leche League, AnotherLook is headquartered in Evanston, Illinois, and Tompson is president and CEO.

The front page of the website states that "the issue of HIV and human milk has been clouded by possibly questionable science, lack of precision concerning the definition of breastfeeding and premature public policy statements." Notwithstanding the fact that evidence of this has existed since 1985, the organization claims to seek evidence that HIV is actually present in breast milk and that it can be transmitted to babies. The Advisory Council of AnotherLook is made up of known AIDS denialists, an alternative-medicine health guru, and a prominent antivaccine doctor who, according to the *Chicago Tribune*, has faced an unusually large number of malpractice lawsuits.

The website also offers position papers that address issues the organization believes are otherwise ignored. Roughly half of AnotherLook's position papers were written by Crowe. His 2001 conference presentation can still be found on the AnotherLook website.

The website also includes presentations on HIV and breastfeeding by other people connected to the denialist movement from other La Leche League conferences—not only in Chicago in 2001, but in San Francisco in 2003, and Chicago in 2005. One such presentation states categorically that HIV has not been detected in human milk and that the chances of being infected with HIV through breastfeeding are between 0 and 0.0001. Another proposes that many children infected with HIV do not die, and that babies infected with HIV through breastfeeding have lower mortality rates than babies infected in utero or at birth. That same paper concludes: "It seems wise to recommend exclusive breastfeeding for at least six months for all women diagnosed as HIV+ . . . even where women can provide replacement feeding that is acceptable, feasible, affordable, sustainable, and safe." Now in her capacity as a UNICEF representative, Labbok was also on that panel, arguing that, since more than 90 percent of women worldwide do not know whether they are infected with HIV, "exclusive breastfeeding should be encouraged for all, for overall child survival."

At the time this panel delivered its recommendations at the 2005 La Leche League International Conference, global health organizations were recommending formula feeding to women who were HIV positive because antiretrovirals were not yet widely available in most countries. In the absence of antiretrovirals, the panel's recommendation would have led to a 15 to 30 percent additional risk of HIV transmission through breastfeeding. The session was also chaired and introduced by Tompson.

Along with Duesberg, the father of AIDS denialism, Tompson is also on the board of Alive and Well AIDS Alternatives, a website founded by AIDS denialist Christine Maggiore. When Maggiore was pregnant with her daughter, Eliza Jane, the parenting magazine *Mothering* published a cover article featuring the pregnant Maggiore urging HIV positive women to "go underground" when they got pregnant, refusing medical care so they could breastfeed and avoid HIV testing for their infants. *Mothering* magazine also honored Tompson with its Living Treasure award in 1998, and as recently as 2013, it published an article by Crowe advising women infected with HIV to tell doctors they are feeding their babies formula while secretly breastfeeding them at home.

Maggiore refused medical treatment for herself and her infant daughter and breastfed her daughter against medical advice. Sadly, Maggiore's three-year-old daughter died of AIDS in 2006, and she herself died of AIDS in 2008. Tompson and Duesberg spoke at her memorial service.

Although Tompson is the breastfeeding advocate who has aligned most visibly with AIDS denialists, she is far from the only one. In fact, when I contacted La Leche League International (LLLI) to ask about its position with respect to Tompson and AnotherLook, I was surprised to learn that Tompson had started her organization "with the blessing of the other League founders." Not only does LLLI "proudly support the work of Marian Tompson," the League spokesperson, Diana West, expressed League support for AnotherLook by explaining that "for over ten years AnotherLook has been the only organization pointing out that there is no evidence supporting the policies that prohibit breastfeeding when a woman is HIV positive." At another point, she explained that Tompson had been moved to start AnotherLook once she realized "that there was no research that proved that a baby born to an HIV positive mother was more likely to get AIDS than a baby fed formula." Not once did West acknowledge that that research had in fact existed for thirty years. Although I had referred to Crowe as a "denialist,"

West called him a "dissident," the insider's term denialists prefer to describe themselves.

Finally, West disclosed that not only does LLLI endorse and support the work of Tompson and AnotherLook, but that many other national and international breastfeeding advocacy organizations do too. As she explained to me, "the International Lactation Consultant Association (ILCA), the US Breastfeeding Committee (USBC), the International Baby Food Action Network (IBFAN), and the National Alliance for Breastfeeding Action (NABA) all greatly respect Marian's work and the work of AnotherLook that helped influence the revision of the WHO and UNICEF breastfeeding recommendations." West concluded by reassuring me that Tompson remains a highly respected leader in the breastfeeding field.

The organizations that West listed pretty much constitute the entire national and international community of breastfeeding advocates, and she was telling me that they all "respect" the work of an organization that claims there is no evidence for the transmission of HIV through breastfeeding. Even after all I had learned about how impassioned lactivists can be, I was completely floored.

LLLI is no longer the tiny fringe organization it was in 1956. It is widely regarded as the largest and most influential breastfeeding advocacy organization in the world. It has local chapters in seventy countries, and more than six thousand accredited leaders worldwide. The organization publishes and distributes hundreds of books and periodicals on breastfeeding. The group is active on Facebook and Twitter, and they have an online web forum. The CDC officially uses "number of La Leche League Leaders per 1,000 live births" as a Breastfeeding Support Indicator to measure how well women are supported with breastfeeding in different parts of the country. The League has consultative status at UNICEF and "affiliate status as part of UNICEF's organizational structure." WHO established "official relations" with LLLI in 1993, in recognition of the important role it plays in promoting breastfeeding. And along with the other organizations West listed above, LLLI is very influential in shaping infant-feeding guidelines around the world.

It's no wonder then that over the course of the last twenty years a major rift has developed between AIDS scientists and the breastfeeding advocacy community. This rift routinely devolves into open hostility at AIDS conferences. Even when they are personally invited, real scientists will not attend workshops and conferences convened by breastfeeding advocates to discuss breastfeeding and HIV/AIDS. Some may fear that attending such conferences would harm their professional reputations. Others are probably simply unwilling to listen to discussions about how the need to make sure children are protected from HIV must be balanced against the need to promote breastfeeding, and that the latter should trump.

AS MEDICAL RESEARCH ADVANCES, WHO has continued to update its recommendations regarding which medications pregnant women should take, when they should start taking them, how long mothers should breastfeed, and under what conditions they should be advised to formula feed. In 2010, it issued new guidelines for infant feeding when mothers are infected with HIV. Those guidelines outline two options. Formula feeding is recommended where formula is "acceptable, feasible, affordable, sustainable, and safe." A combination of breastfeeding and antiretroviral (ARV) treatment is also considered to be an acceptable protocol in countries where formula feeding is not

safe. WHO advises national leaders to assess their own conditions when deciding which option to choose.

This set of recommendations fails to address the question of
what national policy makers should do when formula feeding
is not safe and ARVs are not widely available, which, unfortunately, is still often the case. Some experts estimate that only
37 percent of HIV-infected pregnant women in Africa have
access to ARVs. In much of the world, not much has changed
since 1998 when WHO and UNICEF first changed their infant-
feeding guidelines to recommend formula for babies born to
mothers infected with HIV.

Nevertheless, buried in its 2010 *Guidelines on HIV and Infant Feeding*, WHO addresses this problem by once again recommending breastfeeding. "Even when ARVs are not available,
mothers should be counseled to exclusively breastfeed in the
first six months of life and continue breastfeeding thereafter
unless environmental and social circumstances are safe for, and
supportive of, replacement feeding." WHO has come full circle, resorting to its pre-1998 recommendation that women in
developing countries should breastfeed, regardless of their HIV
status and regardless of their access to ARVs.

This is the victory that West was referring to when she al-
luded to the "revision of the WHO and UNICEF feeding
recommendations." And who could blame her? There is no
question that this new set of recommendations is a victory for
the committed lactivists who campaigned and fought for twelve
long years, from 1998 to 2010, to overturn the guidelines that
recommended formula feeding for women infected with HIV.

Tragically, a closer look at this victory reveals just how hol-
low it is. The contemporary WHO policy was highly influenced
by two studies of infant feeding that discovered that exclusive

breastfeeding for six months reduced the risk of transmission when compared with mixed feeding—a combination of breast and formula feeding. Doctors hypothesize that exclusive breast-feeding better protects the intestinal wall, which acts as a more protective barrier to HIV. Still, the best research has found that even with exclusive breastfeeding there is a 22 percent rate of HIV transmission by six months of age. And as I explained earlier, nowhere in the world does the infant mortality rate approach 22 percent. In Mozambique, a very poor country still wracked with violence and a very poor health-care infrastructure, the infant mortality rate is 9 percent. And the leading cause of infant mortality in Mozambique is malaria, not malnutrition or diarrhea associated with formula feeding.

It's hard to believe that, just as they did from 1985 to 1998, WHO infant-feeding guidelines once again condemn millions of babies to death. The only real difference is that we now have a much more accurate sense of just how many babies contract HIV through breastfeeding.

Even worse, since the discovery that exclusive breastfeeding is better than mixed feeding, evidence has poured in that *exclusive* breastfeeding is not a cultural or historical norm anywhere in the world. Women typically combine breastfeeding with juice, tea, water, or cereals. The women in the study I cited above exclusively breastfed their babies because they were counseled and carefully monitored. Most mothers given the advice to breast-feed exclusively for six months will feed a baby a mixture of breast milk and other liquids and solids. The addition of liquids doubles the risk of HIV transmission through breastfeeding; the addition of solids increases the risk eleven-fold.

Nevertheless, with the momentum of all these recent successes behind them, lactivists have now turned their attention to changing the breastfeeding recommendations for women who are HIV positive in developed countries where formula *is* a safe alternative. Pamela Morrison, an activist with the World Alliance for Breastfeeding Action and a member of the AnotherLook Advisory Council, appears to be leading this crusade. In a number of recent papers and presentations, she has stated that if a mother is on ARVs, the risk of transmitting HIV through breastfeeding is "virtually zero." She uses that figure to support the claim that "IBCLCs can now feel more confident than ever before in supporting HIV positive clients who express a desire to breastfeed."

In fact, researchers estimate that the rate of transmission for mothers on ARVs is between 1 and 5 percent. The most often cited study found that 2.2 percent of women who followed this protocol infected their babies through breastfeeding. Another study put that figure at "less than 1 percent"; 2 of the 709 babies enrolled in the study were infected through breastfeeding. Morrison confirmed to me that it was this latter number she had in mind when she said the rate was "close to zero."

But the conditions under which those "close to zero" transmission rates can be realized are extremely stringent. As Morrison explained to me, they include "full maternal ARV therapy for thirteen weeks prior to delivery; meticulous adherence to medication during pregnancy and breastfeeding; absolutely exclusive breastfeeding for six months; and prompt treatment of any breast/nipple engorgement or abrasions."

Most doctors and public health organizations disagree with Morrison's calculations. Studies have shown that even in the US, pregnant women infected with HIV often fail to take their medication. Not many people have "prompt" access to medical care. Most people would be lucky to get medical attention for engorgement or nipple abrasions in the same week, let alone the same day. If the 2.2 percent figure is correct, one in fifty of the HIV-positive mothers who follow Morrison's advice will infect her baby as a result. If the "less than 1 percent" figure is accurate, that number will, of course, be smaller: 1 in 350 children will be infected.

But many doctors insist that, given the high rates of noncompliance with medication, that number is not easy to reach. They also believe it is still too high, given that formula would eliminate the risk altogether. In countries where formula is a safe alternative, recommending breastfeeding combined with ARV treatment to HIV-infected women simply increases the number of babies who will contract HIV, for no reason other than a fanatical commitment to breastfeeding.

Although HIV transmission is probably the most serious risk associated with breastfeeding, and certainly the one that has had the deadliest consequences, it is not the only one. Mothers can also transmit potentially dangerous levels of toxins, including lead, mercury, and chemicals found in flame retardants, termite poison, and rocket fuel to their babies through breast milk. Babies whose mothers have nutritional deficiencies, which are especially common among vegans and vegetarians, will not get their recommended daily intake of certain important micronutrients from breastfeeding. All breastfed babies are at risk for iron and vitamin D deficiency. Babies with galactosemia, a condition that prevents them from metabolizing a sugar called galactose, will die or become brain damaged if they are breastfed.

The fact is breastfeeding carries risks. It is not universally and indisputably the best choice for all mothers or all babies.

But in their zeal to promote breastfeeding, lactivists seem to have lost sight of the high costs it can impose on babies and mothers. At its most extreme, their zealotry seems to prioritize breastfeeding over the health and well-being, and even the lives, of the babies they are dedicated to protect.

Conclusion

Let's be perfectly clear. The number of women who breast-feed in the United States is very high. Nationwide, 79 percent of women initiate breastfeeding. In New York City, that number was 90 percent, even before the Latch On campaign. Nationwide, 49 percent are still breastfeeding at six months. In 2011, the number of women breastfeeding surpassed the 2010 Healthy People Goals, a target established by the Centers for Disease Control and Prevention (CDC).

	Initiate breast-feeding	Breast-feeding at 6 months	Breast-feeding at 12 months	Exclusive breast-feeding at 6 months
Healthy People Goals 2010	75%	50%	25%	17%
2011 births	79%	49%	27%	19%

Probably the best way to show just how high these numbers are is by comparing the United States to Norway, a country described by the World Health Organization as having "high rates of initiation and duration of breastfeeding." Norway is also a country with generous maternity policies that support breastfeeding. New mothers are entitled to forty-two weeks of maternity leave at full salary, or fifty-two weeks at 80 percent salary. After returning to work, women are entitled to long breaks so they can return home to breastfeed the baby or have the baby brought to work.

	Initiate	Exclusive at 1 week	Exclusive at 3–4 months	Exclusive at 6 months
US[1]	79%	60%	40%	19%
Norway[2]	99%	70%	46%	9%

Clearly, Norway has very high rates of initiation, and it also has high rates of duration—which is to say, a large number of Norwegian women start breastfeeding immediately after giving birth and then continue to do it for a relatively long period of time. At six months, 80 percent of Norwegian babies are still partially breastfeeding. But Norway does not have particularly high rates of exclusive breastfeeding. Even though breastfeeding is a well-established practice in Norway, and even though the country offers one of the most supportive maternity environments in the world, 30 percent of women supplement breast milk with formula by week one of their baby's life. By four months, 54 percent of Norwegian mothers are feeding their babies formula or a combination of formula and breast milk.

The many prominent breastfeeding advocacy campaigns that have emerged in the US in recent years convey the impression that American women are woefully behind when it comes to breastfeeding—that, for one reason or another, they just don't get it. But American breastfeeding rates can only be said to represent failure if we buy into the lactivist refrain that "all women can breastfeed." But as the figures above show, even in Norway not all women can or do breastfeed, and a full 30 percent cannot or do not breastfeed exclusively. By six months, there are actually *more* American mothers exclusively breastfeeding than Norwegian mothers!

There are, in fact, many reasons that women cannot, or should not, breastfeed. The CDC warns that women with HIV/AIDS, hepatitis, tuberculosis, cancer, and other conditions in which the immune system is compromised should not breastfeed. Babies with galactosemia cannot be breastfed. Women who have had breast implants or reductions may not be able to breastfeed, and women who have had mastectomies cannot breastfeed. There are also a number of medications, including many antidepressants, which have not been tested for safety with breastfeeding. Most mothers on those medications would probably be wise to err on the side of caution and avoid breastfeeding.

In the US, the most commonly cited reason for introducing formula is low milk supply. One study found that one in eight women wean early because they are not producing enough milk. The biggest difference between Norway and the United States seems to be that Norwegian women who don't produce enough milk continue breastfeeding and supplement with formula. In the US, they are more likely to stop breastfeeding and switch to formula. Nevertheless, what doctors call lactation failure is undoubtedly a real issue in both countries.

Doctors estimate that up to 15 percent of women suffer from either primary or secondary lactation failure. Sometimes it is caused by a pituitary or thyroid condition. It may also be caused by polycystic ovary syndrome—a condition that leads to hormone imbalances. Complications in childbirth may also affect milk production. Between 5 and 15 percent of women suffer from a condition called hypoplasia, caused by insufficient glandular tissue in the breast. As one breastfeeding advocate explained, "Some moms have been told to 'Just keep trying!' despite telltale signs of insufficient glandular tissue on physical exam, with widely-spaced, tubular breasts and no breast growth during pregnancy." Women with hypoplasia will produce little or no milk. But even though the condition is fairly common, and easy to recognize, it is rarely diagnosed in the United States.

In an article titled "Prevention of Breastfeeding Tragedies," the well-known breastfeeding advocate Dr. Marianne Neifert makes the point that the human body often fails to work "the way it's supposed to." "A health care professional would never tell a diabetic woman that 'every pancreas can make insulin' or insist to a devastated infertility patient that 'every woman can get pregnant.' The fact is that lactation, like all physiologic functions, sometimes fails because of various medical causes." Simply put, not all women produce milk, and not all women produce enough milk to adequately feed their babies. The stubborn refusal to accept this physiological fact can be a form of cruelty.

This same stubborn refusal can put babies at risk as well. A facebook page called Bottle Babies features a thread about hypoplasia, written mostly by women who have been diagnosed with the condition. The thread was started by a woman who was told that "the number of women who cannot breastfeed is insignificant. Almost everyone can breastfeed. You just have to want to." One mother who contributed to the thread told the story of breastfeeding her baby for weeks as he "wasted away in front of" her. Even as the baby endured daily doctor visits

and blood draws, and doctors raised the specter of hospitalization, they also adamantly insisted that she continue exclusive
breastfeeding, and never acknowledged the possibility that the
mother just might not be producing enough milk. She, too, finally learned she had hypoplasia. Her baby was starving.

Comparing breastfeeding rates in the US and Norway is
revealing because the similarities seem to confirm that breastfeeding is *not* possible for every woman. But the differences are
also revealing. The biggest difference between breastfeeding
rates in the US and Norway are at initiation (Norway: 99 percent, US: 79 percent) and at six months (Norway: 80 percent,
US: 50 percent). Norwegian women continue breastfeeding for
much longer than their American counterparts.

At this point, I'm sure the reason for this difference will not be
surprising. The most common reason American women give for
not initiating breastfeeding is that they have to go back to work.
Remember that over 60 percent of US mothers with children under the age of three work, and 30 percent of US mothers take no
maternity leave at all. Those who do take some form of maternity leave know they will be back at work soon, usually within
six weeks. Many probably think, why start, only to be faced with
the potentially agonizing prospect of weaning your infant only
a few weeks later? The lack of maternity leave in the US also explains why American women do not breastfeed as long as their
Norwegian counterparts. Women who return to work are more
than twice as likely to stop breastfeeding than women who have
significant maternity leaves or do not work outside the home. At
six months, most American mothers have already been back at
work for more than four months; Norwegian mothers still have
another four months of maternity leave ahead of them. Taking all
of this into account, an astonishing number of American women
are breastfeeding!

But the fact is, they're doing it at great personal cost. First of all, there are the actual costs associated with a form of infant feeding that is frequently touted as "free." Of course breastfeeding can in fact be mostly free, but in contemporary America, if a mother ever intends to leave the house, it is usually far from it. Here's a back-of-the-envelope calculation of what nursing might cost an average new mother. Many people will spend less, but many others will spend much more.

Cost in purchases if only nursing:

2 nursing tops	$180
2 dresses	$200
1 nightgown	$50
1 tank top	$60
2 nursing bras	$100
1 tube lanolin	$15
15 boxes nursing pads	$100
Nursing pillow	$40
Cover-up	$40
Total:	$785

Additional cost if the mother is pumping (assuming the pump is covered by insurance):

Breast-milk storage bags	$40
Milk tray	$25
4 bottles @ $10 each	$40
Bottle-cleaning equipment	$30
Total:	$135

Additional cost if a mother has any trouble or wants additional support: $400 for lactation consultant visit and follow-up (anywhere from $100 to $350 per hour).

Cost in lost wages over six months for a mother making minimum wage pumping at work (conservative estimate that she is only pumping one hour per day at work): $1,094 @ $8.75 per hour (New York state minimum wage in 2014).

Cost in time over six months: 900 hours of nursing or pumping.

Altogether, these costs add up to $2,414 and 900 hours over six months. At about $600 for six months, formula is quite a bit cheaper. Then there is the expenditure of time; a woman who breastfeeds exclusively for the recommended six months will spend roughly 900 hours doing it: this adds up to 35 hours a week, the equivalent of another full-time job. Which is to say, there's more than one way to do a cost-benefit analysis of breastfeeding.

Most of those we have seen in this book, however, do not appear to take the value of women's time into account. In Chapter 3, I described the cost-benefit analysis that Dr. David Meyers of the AHRQ presented as evidence of the benefits of breastfeeding. He explained that six mothers would have to spend six months breastfeeding to prevent one ear infection. He seemed to think it entirely reasonable that women would spend 5,400 hours breastfeeding to prevent one ear infection, or 15,600 hours breastfeeding to prevent a case of pneumonia. Presented with these numbers, however, even the most devoted parent might well calculate the relative costs and benefits of breastfeeding quite differently than Dr. Meyers. They might also make a different calculation than Melissa Bartick, the lactivist at the Massachusetts Breastfeeding Coalition who calculates that the failure to breastfeed costs the US $13 billion per year, without ever considering the cost that breastfeeding itself imposes—on women.

Breastfeeding also imposes less tangible costs. Women endure enormous pressure to breastfeed not only from other
mothers but from nurses, social workers, and the government.
Many of those who do manage to breastfeed exclusively for at
least six months, as so many large health organizations recommend, pay a significant price, often committing themselves to
a life in which it is understood that their own needs come second, or even third or fourth. These women are giving up jobs
and careers that will be very hard to re-enter years later. They
are growing more financially dependent on husbands at a time
when almost 50 percent of marriages still end in divorce. Or
they are not giving up their jobs but working longer hours for
less pay, under conditions that are demanding and often degrading. They are lugging a heavy breast pump back and forth
to work every day. They are hooking themselves up to that
pump two or three times a day to drain their breasts of milk.
They are enduring ribbing, harassment, and discrimination in
the workplace and long separations from their babies.

If they "fail," as the medical jargon would have it, they suffer
humiliation and guilt. If they are poor, they will be punished
by a government that withholds food from women and infants
who are already at nutritional risk. If they are African American, they will be targeted by a society that has long blamed its
failures on some excluded category of people—as often as not,
African Americans.

As these examples show, the costs of lactivism are not borne
by individuals alone but by our society as a whole. By allowing
some primarily privileged segments of the population to occupy
the moral high ground, the breastfeeding imperative reinforces
race and class discrimination by other means. Whether we realize it or not—and I suspect most people do not—breastfeeding

is an identity marker precisely *because* it is a status symbol. We use breastfeeding to show not only that "we" are good parents, but that other people, especially people who are black, or poor, or unmarried, are not. We are also using it as a way to save money on government food programs. And we are using breastfeeding to restrict women's choices, and to justify interventions into the lives of vulnerable and marginalized women.

We are also using breastfeeding and pumping as a substitute for maternity leave. When women go back to work six weeks after birth, their tiny infants go, most often, to day care. We hope that even though they are separated from their parents for eight to ten hours a day at a very young age, they will be securely attached because they are drinking breast milk. We hope that even though they are exposed to viruses and infections at day care, they will stay healthy because they are drinking breast milk. We hope that even though we are not holding them and talking to them they will meet all the developmental milestones and grow up to be smart and emotionally secure because they are drinking breast milk. And we hope that some of the pain and guilt we feel every morning when we drop them at day care will be alleviated because they are drinking breast milk.

Unfortunately, these hopes are unfounded. Breast milk will not resolve all of the deeply rooted social and structural problems American parents face in trying to raise healthy and secure children. It is no substitute for good and affordable day care close to work or home. It is no substitute for maternity leave. And it is no substitute for accessible and affordable health care.

Our intense focus on breastfeeding as a solution to intractable domestic policy issues needs to be understood as part of the longer US trend toward treating societal well-being as an issue of personal responsibility, a trend that is now most clearly visible in the case of health-care reform. It's not hard to fathom why policy makers and politicians are so deeply invested in promoting breastfeeding, along with healthy eating, exercise, safe sex, and not smoking, as the solution to some of our most enduring and expensive domestic policy problems. As the wrangling that led up to the Obama health-care reforms demonstrated, there really are no good solutions to these problems that are also politically feasible.

By recasting the problem of American health care as a problem of unhealthy and irresponsible individuals, however, public health officials also, of course, play a very significant role in distinguishing between "good" and "bad" citizens. The bad citizens not only bring on their own health problems; they are also responsible for the soaring cost of health care in general. When my friend Todd's mother was diagnosed with lung cancer, he assured me that "she never smoked a day in her life." Over the next two years, as Todd's mother underwent treatment and ultimately died of lung cancer, I would hear him repeat that claim over and over again. He was making sure people knew his mother was not to blame for her horrible illness. A smoker who dies of lung cancer can be dismissed as someone who overtaxes the health-care system through his own selfish or stupid behavior. A nonsmoker is a blameless victim. His mother, Todd made clear, was innocent, worthy of our sympathy.

But the truth is, focusing on individual lifestyle choices in this way doesn't normally cast blame on individuals like Todd's mother—a white, married, upper-middle-class mother and teacher living in the suburbs. The particular lifestyle choices that have come under scrutiny—unsafe sex, smoking, obesity, and the failure to breastfeed—have all been visibly and vociferously linked with particular populations. Unsafe sex is associated with gay men, intravenous drug users, and sex workers. Smoking and obesity are both more prevalent among people who are poor and African American. And it is widely advertised, although somewhat misleading, that breastfeeding is less common among women who are not only poor, African American, and less educated but also unmarried. Over and over again, the habits and conditions that are identified as threatening to public health are habits and conditions that have also been prominently associated with traditionally marginalized and excluded categories of people.

To put this in perspective, it's worth stopping to consider that the CDC website also warns that excessive alcohol use "increases the risk of health problems including injuries, violence, liver diseases, and cancer." In fact, the website features a study reporting that binge drinking costs the United States $223.5 billion per year—significantly more than the estimated $13 billion allegedly associated with the failure to breastfeed. And yet alcohol use has not prompted any major public health initiative or been the subject of a surgeon general's report and (at least since Prohibition) has not been identified as a public health issue. That may be because alcohol use is most common among white men with a household income over $75,000.

The simple fact is that not all potentially dangerous "lifestyle choices" are officially designated as public health issues. The list is in fact highly selective—and tends to exempt habits and conditions that are common among white, male, middle-class, college-educated, heterosexual, married Americans. At the same time, it fosters the impression that this demographic tends to produce good citizens—and now also good parents.

I had a long conversation about this book with an African American cabdriver in Chicago who was driving me to a WIC office in a poor neighborhood on the South Side. I told him that the AAP and the CDC had recently identified breastfeeding as a public health issue, and then I said, "and you'll never guess who they say is not breastfeeding enough . . . " "Black women!" he called out, laughing. Then he added, more ruefully, "What a surprise . . . " To him, the story was so familiar that he'd been a couple of steps ahead of me the whole time.

KNOWING WHAT I KNOW NOW, would I do it all over again?

Well, *yes*. If I was lucky enough, as I have been before, to have a long maternity leave and a baby who latched and thrived, yes, I would breastfeed again. In fact, I wish I *could* do it all over again. As I sit here right now contemplating that question, I'm sorry I'll never have that chance.

But it would be different the next time around. I would have to admit that breastfeeding is not the panacea I brandished so confidently when my children were babies. Even though I might use breastfeeding as a way to feed my baby, I could no longer use it as a talisman to ward off evil. In fact, if we were to make up a list of things that really matter to the well-being of our children, breastfeeding wouldn't even make the top ten.

It's nowhere near as important as loving your child very much and letting her know it. It's not as important as putting your child to sleep on his back, or securely buckling the seatbelt, or finding a good nanny or day care. It's not as important as talking and listening to your child. It's not as important as putting dinner on the table, making sure the crib is safe, keeping an eye on her growth, and building self-confidence. It's not as important as putting a roof over his head. And it's definitely not as important as simply caring, a great deal.

Acknowledgments

This book exists only because of the encouragement and forbearance of many people. I am grateful to the friends I first told about this book—Jenny Nedelsky, Joe Carens, Chloë Atkins, and Aruna Mitra—who urged me to write it, and fast. I am grateful to the friends who read drafts and chapters, Nicoli Nattrass, Mala Htun, Ruth Marshall, and Kate Manson-Smith. I am grateful to the friends who gave me advice along the way, Todd Wiener, Burkhard Bilger, and Joel Bakan. I am grateful for the generosity of the people who agreed to be interviewed for this book. I owe a great debt to our children, Serena, Peter, Riel, and Sam, who have learned more than they ever wanted to know about breastfeeding. I thank my parents, whose love and support have made so many things possible. And I thank my beloved and stoic husband Patrick, who escaped breastfeeding, but could not escape the breastfeeding book.

I am also grateful to Sam Hiyate and Cassandra Rodgers, my agents at The Rights Factory, who bravely took on an author with no blog, no Facebook page, and no Twitter account. And I am grateful to the many wonderful people at Basic Books who brought it all together—Lara Heimert, Liz Dana, Leah Stecher, Melissa Veronesi, Cassie Nelson, and Julie Ford. And none of this would have been even remotely possible without the faith, vision, and persistence of my amazing editor, Alison Mackeen, who believed in this book and made it happen.

Notes

INTRODUCTION

2 **She moved quickly to make the:** Patricia Clark, "Obamacare Encourages Baby Boutiques to Bet on Breast Pumps," *Bloomberg Business Week*, August 26, 2013.

3 **Yummy Mummy now has established relationships:** Telephone interview with Amanda Cole, August 6, 2014.

3 **By the end of the decade:** *Breast Pumps Market (Manual, Single, Double Electric and Hospital Grade Breast Pumps)—Global Industry Analysis, Size, Volume, Share, Growth, Trends and Forecast, 2014–2022.* Transparency Market Research, 2013.

3 **As a new mother in Manhattan:** "Nursing on Cloud Nine," *New York Family*, August 6, 2013.

3 **The store also offers a range of courses:** old.yummymummy store.com/classes.

6 **In 2015, even Pope Francis:** Caroline Bologna, "Pope Francis Welcomes Mothers to Breastfeed in the Sistine Chapel," *The Huffington Post*, January 12, 2015, http://www.huffingtonpost .com/2015/01/12/pope-francis-breastfeeding_n_6456314.html.

6 **Started several years ago:** biglatchon.org.

6 **The advocacy organization:** www.bestforbabes.org/nursing-in -public-hotline-855-nip-free.

7 **Some lactivists have in fact:** Melissa Bartick, "Making the Case: Effective Language for Breastfeeding Advocacy," Massachusetts Breastfeeding Coalition, March 2007, http://massbreastfeeding .org/advocacy/making-the-case/.

7   **Not long ago the supermodel:** Sara Nathan, "Smug Mother
    Gisele Bundchen Says There 'Should Be a Law' Forcing Women
    to Breastfeed for Six Months," *Mail* Online, August 4, 2010.

7   **As Dr. Richard Schanler:** Telephone interview, August 6, 2014.

8   **They breastfeed because:** One blog (http://civileats.com/2011
    /02/22/tea-partiers-milk-anger-over-breastfeeding), for
    example, combines breastfeeding activism with locally grown
    and organic food and sustainable roof gardens.

9   **"a reduction in parental absenteeism":** Melissa Bartick and
    Arnold Reinhold, "The Burden of Suboptimal Breastfeeding in the
    United States: A Pediatric Cost Analysis," *Pediatrics* 125,
    no. 5 (April 2010): e1048–e1056, http://pediatrics.aappublications
    .org/search?author1=Melissa+Bartick&sortspec=date&submit
    =Submit.

9   **Health officials were explicit:** "New York City Health
    Department Launches 'Latch On NYC' Initiative to Support
    Breastfeeding Mothers," New York City Department of Health
    and Mental Hygiene, May 9, 2012, www.nyc.gov/html/doh/html
    /pr2012/pr013-12.shtml.

10 **And, once they start eating:** "The New WIC: Food and Focus
    Breastfeeding," Missouri Department of Health and Senior Services,
    June 2, 2009. This is from a two-page educational handout provided
    to new mothers at WIC clinics in Missouri. The educational
    material was adapted from a similar handout provided in Colorado.
    Health.mo.gov/living/families/.../LWPBFFFoodPkgEducation.doc.

10 **Evidence that breastfeeding can transmit HIV:** John B. Ziegler
    et al., "Postnatal Transmission of AIDS-Associated Retrovirus
    from Mother to Infant," *The Lancet* 325, no. 8434 (April 1985):
    896–898.

10 **But global public health officials:** Edith White, *Breastfeeding and
    HIV/AIDS: The Research, the Politics, the Women's Responses*
    (Jefferson, NC: McFarland, 1999).

10 **When organizations like the World Health:** www.anotherlook
    .org/presentations.php.

10 **In Chapter 7, I describe:** E-mail exchange with Diana West,
    La Leche League International (LLLI) media contact and
    spokesperson, April 2015.

11 **Yet the fact is that:** "More Mothers Are Breastfeeding: African
    American Mothers Need More Support," Centers for Disease

Control and Prevention, Department of Health and Human
Services, www.cdc.gov/media/releases/2013/p0207_breast
_feeding.html.

11 **But it is also true that:** For 2007 data, see "Provisional Breast-
feeding Rates by Socio-demographic Factors, Among Children
Born in 2007 (Percent +/–half 95% Confidence Interval),"
National Immunization Survey, Centers for Disease Control
and Prevention (CDC), Department of Health and Human
Services (HHS), www.cdc.gov/breastfeeding/data/NIS_data
/2007/socio-demographic_any.htm. For 2010 data, see "Rates of
Any and Exclusive Breastfeeding by Socio-demographics
Among Children Born in 2010 (Percentage +/-half 95%
Confidence Interval)," National Immunization Survey, CDC,
HHS, www.cdc.gov/breastfeeding/data/nis_data/rates-any
-exclusive-bf-socio-dem-2010.htm.

12 **"So that it's not just:** Sarah Maslin, "Helping Hands Also
Expose NY Divide," *New York Times*, November 16, 2012.

13 **"to provide reasonable break time":** www.ncsl.org/issues
-research/health/breastfeeding-state-laws.aspx.

13 **But fully 30 percent of them:** US Department of Health and
Human Services (HHS), Health Resources and Services
Administration, Maternal and Child Health Bureau, *Women's
Health USA 2011* (Rockville, MD: HHS, 2011), www.mchb.hrsa
.gov/whusa11/hstat/hsrmh/pages/233ml.html.

14 **Over the last decade in particular:** Michael Johnsen, "Breast
feeding Grows into Destination Category," *Drug Store News* 30,
no. 6 (May 19, 2008): 52.

14 **Many leading physicians and researchers:** Interview with Dr.
Thomas Farley, August 5, 2014, New York City; interview with
Dr. Michael Kramer, December 12, 2013, Montreal, Canada.

14 **A company called Prolacta:** Andrew Pollack, "Breast Milk
Becomes a Commodity, with Mothers Caught Up in Debate,"
New York Times, March 20, 2015.

15 **He served it crusted:** www.dailymail.co.uk/news/article
-1256200/Daniel-Angerers-breast-milk-cheese-sale-chef-s
-Klee-Brasserie-New-York.html.

20 **A few years later, after I had stopped:** Hanna Rosin, "The Case
Against Breast-Feeding," *The Atlantic*, April 2009.

CHAPTER 1

27 **Ancient documemts also show:** Emily E. Stevens et al., "A History of Infant Feeding," *Journal of Perinatal Education* 18, no. 2 (spring 2009): 32–39.

27 **As early as 950 BC:** Ibid.

28 **A Boston study from the early 1900s:** Jacqueline H. Wolf, "Public Health Then and Now," *American Journal of Public Health* 93, no. 12 (December 2003): 2001.

29 **In 1912, only 39 percent:** Ibid., 2003.

29 **The range of choices seemed:** Ibid., 2002.

29 **They often instructed mothers:** Lynn Y. Weiner, "Reconstructing Motherhood: The La Leche League in Postwar America," *Journal of American History* 80, no. 4 (March 1994): 1365–1366.

30 **From that initial meeting of seven friends:** Ibid., 1359.

31 **Historians have argued that:** Christina G. Bobel, "Bounded Liberation: A Focused Study of La Leche League International," *Gender and Society* 15, no. 1 (February 2001): 135.

31 **"We weren't encouraged to ask questions:** Molly M. Ginty, *"Our Bodies, Ourselves Turns* 35 Today," Women's eNews, May 2004, http://womensenews.org/story/health/040504/our-bodies -ourselves-turns-35-today.

32 **It simply recommends calling:** Boston Women's Health Collective, *Women and Their Bodies: A Course,* 1970, 175, www.ourbodiesourselves.org/cms/assets/uploads/2014/04 /Women-and-Their-Bodies-1970.pdf.

32 **In an era when women devoured:** Bobel, "Bounded Liberation," 140.

33 **"I think we're being two-faced:** Mary Ann Cahill, *Seven Voices, One Dream* (Schaumburg, IL: La Leche League International, 2001), 151.

34 **Although she received a standing:** Ibid., 133–134.

34 **"Our plea to any mother:** Linda M. Blum and Elizabeth A. Vandewater, "Mother to Mother: A Maternalist Organization in Late Capitalist America," *Social Problems* 40, no. 3 (August 1993): 288; quoted from La Leche League International, *The Womanly Art of Breastfeeding* (Franklin Park, IL: La Leche League International, 1981) 271.

35 **In 1971, the nadir of American breastfeeding:** "Ross Labs Breastfeeding Statistics," KellyMom, http://kellymom.com/fun /trivia/ross-data/.

37　**She told me she was drawn:** Blum and Vandewater, "Mother to Mother," 300; Bobel, "Bounded Liberation," 146.

38　**Most of those deaths were in Africa:** Ramon Martinez, "A Global Overview of the Magnitude, Disparities and Trend of Infant Mortality in the World: 1950–2011," Health Intelligence, March 2013, http://healthintelligence.drupalgardens.com /content/global-overview-magnitude-disparities-and-trend -infant-mortality-world-1950-2011.

38　**In the Soviet Union:** Christopher Davis and Murray Feshbach, *Rising Infant Mortality in the USSR in the 1970s,* Series P-95, No. 74 (Washington, DC: US Bureau of Census, September 1980).

38　**Malaria, measles, injury:** Kathryn M. Andrews et al., "Mortality, Infant," in Marshall M. Haith and Janette B. Benson, eds., *Encyclopedia of Infant and Early Childhood Development* (Waltham, MA: Academic Press, 2008), 343–359.

38　**But in Africa and Southeast Asia:** Ibid.

39　**Nestlé expanded by leaps:** Lauren Pomerantz, "Death, Diarrhea, and Developing Nations: Nestlé and the Ethics of Infant Formula," TeachSpace, summer 2001, www.teachspace.org /personal/research/nestle/title.html. Pomerantz also notes that "by 1977, Nestlé had 81 plants in 27 non-industrialized countries, and 728 sales centers in all parts of the world."

39　**Nestlé commanded a 50 percent share:** Stephen Solomon, "The Controversy over Infant Formula," *New York Times,* December 6, 1981, 1–6, www.nytimes.com/1981/12/06 /magazine/the-controversy-over-infant-formula.html.

39　**In Brazil, formula was:** Ibid., 6.

39　**"When one considers that for every:** Ibid.

40　**As they helped mothers cope:** Ibid.

40　**But health officials nonetheless:** Pomerantz, "Death, Diarrhea, and Developing Nations."

40　**In a 1981 *New York Times* article:** Solomon, "The Controversy over Infant Formula," 6.

41　**In 1979, researchers in Indonesia:** Ibid.

41　**It could consume 30 to 50 percent:** Joanna Moorhead, "Milking It," *The Guardian,* May 15, 2007, www.theguardian.com/business /2007/may/15/medicineandhealth.lifeandhealth.

41　**One study conducted in Indonesia:** Solomon, "The Controversy over Infant Formula," 6.

41　**A doctor in Bangladesh explained:** Moorhead, "Milking It."

41 **A Jamaican mother who brought:** Solomon, "The Controversy over Infant Formula."

41 **"Stored at room temperature:** Ibid.

42 **His pamphlet went beyond:** Mike Muller, "The Baby Killer: A War on Want Investigation into the Promotion and Sale of Powdered Baby Milks in the Third World," War on Want, London, March 1974.

43 **"of course it was a slam dunk!:** Interview with Edith White Fletcher, September 19, 2014.

44 **"Typically, they were in their:** Ibid.

44 **"The client might be a woman:** Ibid.

46 **Amazingly, it has been in place ever since:** Anwar Fazal, "Message to IBFAN's 30th Anniversary on 12 Oct 2009," IBFAN, 2009, www.ibfan.org/art/Anwar_Fazal_-_message_to_IBFAN %27s_30th1.pdf. Further, according to an online poll conducted in 2005, Nestlé is among the top four most boycotted companies in the world. See Ian Johnston, "Nestlé: The World's Biggest Food Company and One of the 'Most Boycotted,'" *London Telegraph*, September 2009, www.telegraph.co.uk/news /worldnews/africaandindianocean/zimbabwe/6235566/Nestle -the-worlds-biggest-food-company-and-one-of-the-most -boycotted.html.

CHAPTER 2

51 **The second wave was triggered:** Betty Friedan, *The Feminine Mystique* (New York: W. W. Norton, 1963).

52 **Steinem focused on issues that highlighted:** Keri Philips, "Second Wave Feminism," *ABC Radio National*, October 13, 2013. Transcript and audio recording of interview available online: www.abc.net.au/radionational/programs/rearvision /second-wave-feminism/4983136#transcript.

55 **"Chances are also good that, consciously or not:** Kate Pickert, "The Man Who Remade Motherhood," *Time*, May 21, 2012.

57 **Mothers who practice attachment:** Ibid.

58 **As children grow up:** Elizabeth Pantley, *The No-Cry Sleep Solution for Toddlers and Preschoolers: Gentle Ways to Stop Bedtime Battles and Improve Your Child's Sleep* (New York: McGraw-Hill, 2005).

58 **The parents in the *Time* magazine article:** Pickert, "The Man Who Remade Motherhood."

60 **The French philosopher and feminist:** Elisabeth Badinter, *The Conflict: How Modern Motherhood Undermines the Status of Women* (New York: Metropolitan Books, 2011).

60 **Blogger and feminist Jessica Valenti's:** Jessica Valenti, *Why Have Kids? A New Mom Explores the Truth About Parenting and Happiness* (Boston: Houghton Mifflin Harcourt, 2012); Ayelet Waldman, *Bad Mother: A Chronicle of Maternal Crimes, Minor Calamities, and Occasional Moments of Grace* (New York: Doubleday, 2009).

60 **Working moms feel even worse:** Leslie Morgan Steiner, ed., *Mommy Wars: Stay-at-Home and Career Moms Face Off on Their Choices, Their Lives, Their Families* (New York: Random House, 2007).

63 **But they are also challenging:** "Animal Feed," GRACE Communications Foundation, www.sustainabletable.org/260/animal-feed.

64 **The term *fair trade* is a critique:** Adam Carlson, "Are Consumers Willing to Pay More for Fair Trade Certified Coffee?" accessed October 2013, http://economics.nd.edu/assets/31977/carlson_bernoulli.pdf; see also "Coffee," Fairtrade Canada, http://fairtrade.ca/en/products/coffee-0.

64 **Local food movements are prominent:** Deloitte, *Best Practices in Local Food: A Guide for Municipalities*, Ontario Municipal Knowledge Network and Association of Municipalities of Ontario, www.roma.on.ca/ROMA-Docs/Reports/2013BestPracticesinLocalFoodAGuideforMunicipalitie.aspx.

64 **In fact *The Surgeon General's*:** US Department of Health and Human Services (HHS), *The Surgeon General's Call to Action to Support Breastfeeding* (Washington, DC: HHS, Office of the Surgeon General, 2011).

64 **Mother Nature Network (www.mnn.com):** Jennifer Chait, "6 Green Reasons Why Breastfeeding Is the Best Feeding," Mother Nature Network, August 1, 2009, www.mnn.com/family/family-activities/stories/6-green-reasons-why-breastfeeding-is-the-best-feeding.

65 **Another organization dedicated:** Cherise Udell, "Breastfeeding Is an Environmental Issue," Care2, May 9, 2013, www.care2.com/greenliving/breastfeeding-is-an-environmental-issue.html.

65 **"After all," says one activist:** Jill Fehrenbacher, "Chef Daniel Angerer Defends Cheese Made from Wife's Breast Milk,"

Inhabitat, March 9, 2010, http://inhabitat.com/chef-daniel
-angerer-defends-cheese-made-from-wife's-breast-milk.

65   **As one self-identified environmentalist:** Udell, "Breastfeeding
Is an Environmental Issue."

66   **They advise mothers who:** For example, see Bess Bedell, "Biblical
Breastfeeding," A Warrior Mom (blog), August 12, 2012, https://
awarriormom.wordpress.com/2012/12/09/biblical-breastfeeding/.

66   **In a quick twenty minutes on Google:** Nancy Campbell,
"Breastfeeding God's Way," Above Rubies, accessed: October
2013, www.aboverubies.org/index.php/component/content
/article?id=322; Marsha Bearden, "What God Says About
Breastfeeding," Mothering from the Heart, accessed March 5,
2012, http://motheringfromtheheart.com/whatgod.htm.

67   **Bingham offers various pieces:** Heidi Bingham, "Breastfeeding
by Design: Part 1," *Cornerstone*, 1998, www.internetarchaeology
.org/y2k/1989/famtopics/brfding.html.

67   **Breastfeeding satisfies not only:** "Breastfeeding," Gentle
Christian Mothers, www.gentlechristianmothers.com/topics
/breastfeeding.php.

67   **Whereas these mothers are using:** Rex D. Russell, "Design in
Infant Nutrition," *Acts & Facts* 24, no. 1 (1995), www.icr.org
/article/design-infant-nutrition.

68   **He concludes, "Is there any way . . . Thank the Creator!":** Ibid.

68   **"The husband has the final authority:** Bingham, "Family
Topics."

68   **Christian roles are firmly rooted:** S. Michael Houdmann, "How
Does the Bible Define a Good Christian Family?" Got Questions
Ministries, accessed: October 2013, www.gotquestions.org
/Christian-family.html.

68   **"God's plan for women:** Campbell, "Breastfeeding God's Way."

68   **"If it's on your mind, ask yourself:** Bingham, "Breastfeeding by
Design: Part 1."

68   **"The rejection in our hearts:** Campbell, "Breastfeeding God's
Way."

68   **Part of the reason so many:** Lauren Markoe, "Breastfeeding Is on
the Rise but in Church It's Still an Issue," *Religion News Service*,
January 2, 2014; Rachel Marie Stone, "Breast-Feeding in the Back
Pew: Why Are We So Uncomfortable When Nursing Mothers

Imitate God in Church?" *Christianity Today*, December 12, 2012;
Jennifer Laycock, "Mistaken Attitudes About Breastfeeding in
Public," The Lactivist Blog, November 30, 2005, http://thelactivist
.blogspot.ca/2005/11/mistaken-attitudes-about-breastfeeding.html.
69 **He also told reporters:** Mandy Velez, "Pope Francis Supports
Breastfeeding Enough to Know It Needs to Happen in Public,"
Huffington Post, December 18, 2013, www.huffingtonpost
.com/2013/12/18/pope-francis-supports-breastfeeding-moms
_n_4467719.html.
69 **God did it right the first time:** Bedell, "Biblical Breastfeeding."
69 **If God provided mothers:** Ibid.
69 **"For me, breastfeeding was not:** Ibid.

CHAPTER 3

73 **He authored the very influential:** Michael S. Kramer and
Ritsuko Kakuma, *The Optimal Duration of Exclusive
Breastfeeding: A Systematic Review* (Geneva, Switzerland:
WHO, 2002).
74 **According to Buyken, there is:** Annette E. Buyken et al.,
"Effects of Breastfeeding on Health Outcomes in Childhood:
Beyond Dose-Response Relations," *American Journal of Clinical
Nutrition* 87, no. 6 (June 2008): 1964.
78 **At that point, there were well over:** Anne L. Wright and
Richard J. Schanler, "The Resurgence of Breastfeeding at the End
of the Second Millennium," *Journal of Nutrition* 131, no. 2
(February 2001): 4215–4255.
80 **Although most mothers in both groups:** Michael S. Kramer,
"Methodological Challenges in Studying Long-Term Effects of
Breast-Feeding," in Gail Goldberg et al., eds., *Breast-Feeding:
Early Influences on Later Health* (New York: Springer Science,
2009), 130–132.
80 **In a *JAMA* assessment of the study:** Ruth A. Lawrence,
"Breastfeeding in Belarus," *Journal of American Medical
Association* 285, no. 4 (January 2001): 463–464.
82 **One study often cited:** Aviva Mimouni-Bloch et al.,
"Breastfeeding May Protect from Developing Attention-Deficit
/Hyperactivity Disorder," *Breastfeeding Medicine* 8, no. 4 (August
2013): 363–367.

82 **A number of meta-analyses:** Ip et al. for example concluded that "there were insufficient good quality data to address the relationship between breastfeeding and cardiovascular diseases and infant mortality." See Stanley Ip et al., "Breastfeeding and Maternal and Infant Health Outcomes in Developed Countries," *Evidence Report/Technology Assessment No. 153* (Rockville, MD: AHRQ, April 2007).

82 **Between 1990 and 2007:** "How Science Goes Wrong: Scientific Research Has Changed the World, Now It Needs to Change Itself," *The Economist*, October 19, 2013, http://www.economist .com/news/leaders/21588069-scientific-research-has-changed -world-now-it-needs-change-itself-how-science-goes-wrong.

83 **Scientists have expressed concern:** Christopher G. Owen et al., "The Effect of Breastfeeding on Mean Body Mass Index Throughout Life: A Quantitative Review of Published and Unpublished Observational Evidence," *American Journal of Clinical Nutrition* 82, no. 6 (December 2005): 1298–1307.

83 **And it's not just that the list:** "7 Ways Breastfed Babies Become Healthier Adults," AskDrSears, accessed December 2013, http:// www.askdrsears.com/topics/breastfeeding/why-breast-best /7-ways-breastfed-babies-become-healthier-adults.

83 **It's that everyone has a different list:** Moises Velasquez-Manoff, "Who Has the Guts for Gluten?" *New York Times*, Opinion Pages, February 24, 2013, www.nytimes.com/2013/02/24/opinion /sunday/what-really-causes-celiac-disease.html.

83 **"Now that science has beaten back:** Anemona Hartocollis, "Running for Your Life," *New York Times*, November 5, 2010, www.nytimes.com/2010/11/07/nyregion/07farley.html.

84 **But compared to other breastfeeding:** "New York City Health Department Launches 'Latch On NYC' Initiative to Support Breastfeeding Mothers," New York City Department of Health and Mental Hygiene, May 9, 2012, www.nyc.gov/html/doh/html /pr2012/pr013-12.shtml.

84 **he didn't feel comfortable:** Interview with Dr. Thomas Farley, August 5, 2014, New York City.

84 **The initial results of the PROBIT study:** Michael S. Kramer et al., "Promotion of Breastfeeding Intervention Trial (PROBIT): A Randomized Trial in the Republic of Belarus," *Journal of American Medical Association* 285, no. 4 (January 2001): 417.

84 **By following up with babies breastfed:** Michael S. Kramer et al., "Infant Growth and Health Outcomes Associated with 3

Compared with 6 Mo of Exclusive Breastfeeding," *American Journal for Clinical Nutrition* 78, no. 2 (August 2003): 294.

85 **On the other hand, the PROBIT:** Kramer et al., "Promotion of Breastfeeding Intervention Trial," 413.

85 **"We can see in vitro . . . worked out":** Interview with Kramer, December 12, 2013.

85 **Milk oligosaccharides and lactoferrin:** Thierry Hennet et al., "Decoding Breast Milk Oligosaccharides," *Swiss Medical Weekly* 144 (February 14, 2014); J. H. Brock, "Lactoferrin in Human Milk: Its Role in Iron Absorption and Protection Against Enteric Infection in the Newborn Infant," *Archives of Disease in Childhood* 55, no. 6 (June 1980): 417–421; "Lactoferrin," WebMD, 2009, www.webmd.com/vitamins-supplements /ingredientmono-49-lactoferrin.aspx?activeingredientid=49& activeingredientname=lactoferrin.

85 **Ruth Lawrence, the editor of the journal:** David Meyers, "Breastfeeding and Health Outcomes," *Breastfeeding Medicine* 4, no. S1 (October 2009): S13.

86 **According to Meyers, "the evidence suggests:** Ibid.

86 **"At least 26 infants will have:** Ip et al., "Breastfeeding and Maternal and Infant Health," 40.

86 **The AHRQ meta-analysis:** Ibid., 6.

86 **Based on that assessment, many neonatal:** Jae H. Kim et al., "Challenges in the Practice of Human Milk Nutrition in the Neonatal Intensive Care Unit," *Early Human Development* 89, Suppl. 2 (2013): S35–S38; Sandra Sullivan et al., "An Exclusively Human Milk–Based Diet Is Associated with a Lower Rate of Necrotizing Enterocolitis Than a Diet of Human Milk and Bovine Milk-Based Products," *Journal of Pediatrics* 156, no. 4 (December 28, 2009): 562–567.

87 **The initial PROBIT study corroborated:** Kramer et al., "Promotion of Breastfeeding Intervention Trial," 413–420.

87 **A PROBIT follow-up study:** Michael S. Kramer et al., "Effect of Prolonged and Exclusive Breast Feeding on Risk of Allergy and Asthma: Cluster Randomised Trial," *British Medical Journal* 335, no. 7624 (2007): 4.

88 **At that point, the task force reported:** American Academy of Pediatrics, "The Changing Concept of Sudden Infant Death Syndrome: Diagnostic Coding Shifts, Controversies Regarding the Sleeping Environment, and New Variables to Consider in Reducing Risk," *Pediatrics* 116, no. 5 (November 2005):

1245–1255; see also Alison Steube, "The Risks of Not Breastfeeding for Mothers and Infants," *Review in Obstetrics and Gynecology* 2, no. 4 (Fall 2009): 222–213.

88 **Another task force reaffirmed that:** http://stats.org/stories/2011/breastfeeding_risk_sids_jul11.html. Source material available in print from author.

88 **In 2011, however:** "SIDS and Other Sleep-Related Infant Deaths: Expansion of Recommendations for a Safe Infant Sleeping Environment," *Pediatrics* (2011) 128: 1030–1039.

88 **The following year, a task force:** E. A. Mitchell et al., "Scientific Consensus Forum to Review the Evidence Underpinning the Recommendations of the Australian SIDS and Kids Safe Sleeping Health Promotion Programme," *Journal of Pediatric Child Health* 48 (October 2012): 626–633.

88 **A subsequent meta-analysis concluded:** F. R. Hauck et al., "Breastfeeding and Reduced Risk of Sudden Infant Death Syndrome: A Meta-Analysis," *Pediatrics* 128 (2011): 103–110.

89 **the AHRQ meta-analysis:** Stanley Ip et al., "A Summary of the Agency for Healthcare Research and Quality's Evidence Report on Breastfeeding in Developed Countries," *Breastfeeding Medicine* 4, no. 1 (2009): 6.

89 **On the other hand, research:** Linda Ferrante and Siri Hauge Opdal, "Sudden Infant Death Syndrome and the Genetics of Inflammation," *Frontiers in Immunology*, February 20, 2015, www.ncbi.nlm.nih.gov/pmc/articles/PMC4335605/.

89 **In some, though clearly not all cases:** Mohammad Alfelali and Gulam Khandaker, "Infectious Causes of Sudden Infant Death Syndrome," *Pediatric Respiratory Reviews* 15 (2014): 307–311.

89 **"Yes, we did consider . . . was pretty shaky":** Interview with Farley, August 5, 2014.

89 **The list did not include SIDS:** www2.aap.org/breastfeeding/policyonbreastfeedinganduseofhumanmilk.html.

89 **Six of the remaining seven studies:** Christopher G. Owen et al., "Does Breastfeeding Influence Risk of Type 2 Diabetes in Later Life? A Quantitative Analysis of Published Evidence," *American Journal of Clinical Nutrition* 84, no. 5 (November 2006): 1043–1054.

90 **But only three of those studies:** Ibid.

90 **If there is, they estimate that:** Ibid.

90 **This means that the risk:** www.stats.org/stories/2011/Breast feeding_leukemia_nov11_11.html. Source material available in print from author.

90 **The overall conclusion of the AHRQ:** Jeanne-Marie Guise et al., "Review of Case Controlled Studies Related to Breastfeeding and Reduced Risk of Childhood Leukemia," *Pediatrics* 116, no. 5 (November 2005): 724–731.

91 **The authors of that study:** Richard M. Martin et al., "Breast-Feeding and Childhood Cancer: A Systematic Review with Metaanalysis," *International Journal of Cancer* 117, no. 6 (December 2005): 1020–1031.

91 **Although some studies have:** Steube, "The Risks of Not Breastfeeding for Mothers and Infants," 224.

91 **Another meta-analysis reported that:** Eyal Klement et al., "Breastfeeding and Risk of Inflammatory Bowel Disease: A Systematic Review with Meta-Analysis," *American Journal of Clinical Nutrition* 80, no. 5 (November 2004): 1342–1352.

91 **It's unlikely that breastfeeding:** Interview with Kramer, December 12, 2013.

91 **And although a small Israeli:** Mimouni-Bloch et al., "Breastfeeding May Protect from Developing Attention-Deficit /Hyperactivity Disorder."

91 **the PROBIT study found:** Kramer et al., "Effect of Prolonged and Exclusive Breast Feeding."

91 **Ultimately, however, Kramer cautioned:** Michael S. Kramer et al., "Breastfeeding and Child Cognitive Development: New Evidence from a Large Randomized Trial," *Journal of the American Medical Association* 65, no. 5 (May 2008): 582; Erik L. Mortensen et al., "The Association Between Duration of Breastfeeding and Adult Intelligence," *Journal of the American Medical Association* 287, no. 22 (May 2002): 2365–2371.

91 **Basically, he says "we shouldn't:** Interview with Kramer, December 12, 2013. In the article reporting the results, he explained seven points are "not the difference between a genius and a mentally retarded child." Molly Edmonds, "Does Breastfeeding Make Better Babies?" HowStuffWorks, 2013, http://health.howstuffworks.com/pregnancy-and-parenting /baby-health/baby-care/breast-feeding-better.htm/printable.

92 **Those systematic variations:** Interview with Kramer, December 12, 2013.

92   **There is disagreement over whether:** James W. Anderson et al.,
     "Breast-Feeding and Cognitive Development: A Meta-Analysis,"
     American Journal of Clinical Nutrition 70, no. 4 (October 1999):
     525–535; Anjali Jain et al., "How Good Is the Evidence Linking
     Breastfeeding and Intelligence?" *Pediatrics* 109, no. 6 (June
     2002): 1044–1053.

93   **A recent Brazilian study that:** Cesar G. Victora et al.,
     "Association Between Breastfeeding and Intelligence,
     Educational Attainment, and Income at 30 Years of Age: A
     Prospective Birth Cohort Study from Brazil," *The Lancet* 3, no. 4
     (April 2015): e199–e205.

93   **But two prominent studies that:** Geoff Der et al., "Effect of
     Breast Feeding on Intelligence in Children: Prospective Study,
     Sibling Pairs Analysis, and Meta-Analysis," *British Medical
     Journal* 333, no. 945 (November 2006); Cynthia G. Colen and
     David M. Ramey, "Is Breast Truly Best? Estimating the Effects of
     Breastfeeding on Long-Term Child Health and Wellbeing in the
     United States Using Sibling Comparisons," *Social Science &
     Medicine* 109 (May 2014): 55–65.

93   **The AHRQ meta-analysis:** Ip et al., "A Summary of the Agency
     for Healthcare Research," S17.

93   **Recent research and reviews:** Richard M. Martin et al., "Effects
     of Promoting Longer-Term and Exclusive Breastfeeding on
     Adiposity and Insulin-Like Growth Factor-I at Age 11.5 Years: A
     Randomized Trial," *Journal of the American Medical Association*
     309, no. 10 (March 2013): 1005–1013; Christopher G. Owen et
     al., "Effect of Breast Feeding in Infancy on Blood Pressure in
     Later Life: Systematic Review and Meta-Analysis," *British
     Medical Journal* 327, no. 7425 (November 2003): 1; Michael S.
     Kramer et al., "The Effect of Prolonged and Exclusive Breast-
     Feeding on Dental Caries in Early School Age Children," *Caries
     Research* 41, no. 6 (2007): 484–488.

93   **But studies that used infant-feeding records:** Ip et al., "A
     Summary of the Agency for Healthcare Research," S24.

93   **A 2003 study published:** Anette-G. Ziegler et al., "Early Infant
     Feeding and Risk of Developing Type 1 Diabetes–Associated
     Autoantibodies," *Journal of the American Medical Association*
     290, no. 13 (November 2003): 1721–1728. Another 2009
     meta-analysis reported simply that the results of research on
     a link between breastfeeding and type 1 diabetes has been

"mixed": see Steube, "The Risks of Not Breastfeeding for Mothers and Infants," 225.

93 **The AHRQ meta-analysis also:** Martin et al., "Breast-Feeding and Childhood Cancer."

94 **In the last few years:** Malena Amusa, "Michelle Obama Urged to Speak Out for Breastfeeding," WeNews, February 8, 2010, www.doulas.com/m/news/view/Michelle-Obama-speaks-about -Breastfeeding.

94 **But the fact remains that a number:** Cesar G. Victora et al., "Anthropometry and Body Composition of 18 Year Old Men According to Duration of Breast Feeding: Birth Cohort Study from Brazil," *British Medical Journal* 327, no. 7240 (October 16, 2003); L. Li et al., "Breast Feeding and Obesity in Childhood: Cross Sectional Study," *British Medical Journal* 327, no. 7240 (October 16, 2003); Christopher G. Owen et al., "Effect of Infant Feeding on the Risk of Obesity Across the Life Course: A Quantitative Review of Published Evidence," *Pediatrics* 115, no. 5 (May 1, 2005): 1367–1377; Michael S. Kramer et al., "Effects of Prolonged and Exclusive Breastfeeding on Child Height, Weight, Adiposity, and Blood Pressure at Age 6.5 y: Evidence from a Large Randomized Trial," *Americal Journal of Clinical Nutrition* 86, no. 6 (December 2007): 1717–1721; Mohammadreza Vafa et al., "Relationship Between Breastfeeding and Obesity in Childhood," *Journal of Health, Population, and Nutrition* 30, no. 3 (September 2012): 303–310; Richard M. Martin et al., "Effects of Promoting Longer-Term and Exclusive Breastfeeding on Adiposity and Insulin-Like Growth Factor-I at Age 11.5 Years: A Randomized Trial," *Journal of the American Medical Association* 309, no. 10 (March 2013): 1005–1013; Colen and Ramey, "Is Breast Truly Best?"

49 **Kramer believes this is what:** Interview with Kramer, December 12, 2013.

CHAPTER 4

98 **That was when the:** Arthur I. Eidelman and Richard J. Schanler, "Breastfeeding and the Use of Human Milk," *Pediatrics* 129, no. 3 (February 2012): e827.

98 **Media outlets including *Time*:** Bonnie Rochman, "Why Pediatricians Say Breast-Feeding Is About Public Health, Not

Just Lifestyle," *Time*, February 29, 2012, http://healthland.time
.com/2012/02/29/why-pediatricians-say-breast-feeding-is-about
-public-health-not-just-lifestyle.

99   **"In framing it that way:** Ibid.

99   **"It's not should I or:** Ibid.

99   **That workshop was held:** Ruth Lawrence is the editor of
Breastfeeding Medicine, a highly respected breastfeeding advocate, and the doctor who has consistently stood behind the
results of the PROBIT study, reported in Chapter 2, which has
generally found very modest or nonexistent benefits associated
with breastfeeding.

99   **"Breastfeeding is believed:** Anthony Waddell, ed., "Report of
the Surgeon General's Workshop on Breastfeeding & Human
Lactation," US Department of Health and Human Services, June
1984, 1, http://profiles.nlm.nih.gov/NN/B/C/G/F.

100   **The blueprint urged doctors:** Jacqueline H. Wolf, "Low
Breastfeeding Rates and Public Health in the United States,"
American Journal of Public Health 93, no. 12 (December 2003):
2000–2010.

100   **In so doing, Benjamin managed:** US Department of Health
and Human Services (HHS), *The Surgeon General's Call to
Action to Support Breastfeeding* (Washington, DC: HHS, Office
of the Surgeon General, 2011), v, www.cdc.gov/breastfeeding
/promotion/calltoaction.htm.

100   **"Better infant health means:** Ibid., 3.

100   **The surgeon general explained:** Ibid., 54.

101   **She advises lactivists to counter:** Melissa Bartick, "Making the
Case: Effective Language for Breastfeeding Advocacy,"
Massachusetts Breastfeeding Coalition, March 2007, http://mass
breastfeeding.org/advocacy/making-the-case.

101   **As the essay continues:** Ibid.

102   **She and an IT consultant named:** Melissa Bartick and Arnold
Reinhold, "The Burden of Suboptimal Breastfeeding in the United
States: A Pediatric Cost Analysis," *Pediatrics* 125, no. 5 (April
2010): e1048–e1056, http://pediatrics.aappublications.org
/search?author1=Melissa+Bartick&sortspec=date&submit
=Submit.

102   **"If 90% of US families could:** Ibid., e1048.

102   **"almost all the data . . . represent causality":** HHS, *The Surgeon
General's Call to Action*, 2.

103   **Finally, Bartick reached the astonishing sum:** For a scathing critique of Bartick's so-called study, see www.stats.org/stories /2011/Breastfeeding_leukemia_nov11_11.html. Source material available in print from author.

104   **"Well, how do *you* . . . well-respected studies":** Telephone interview with Dr. Richard Schanler, August 6, 2014.

105   **The AHRQ meta-analysis identified:** Stanley Ip et al., "Breastfeeding and Maternal and Infant Health Outcomes in Developed Countries" *Evidence Report/Technology Assessment No. 153* (Rockville, MD: Agency for Healthcare Research and Quality, April 2007), 5.

105   **Drawing on other research:** Eidelman and Schanler, "Breastfeeding and the Use of Human Milk," e830.

105   **The AHRQ meta-analysis concluded:** Ip et al., "Breastfeeding and Maternal and Infant Health Outcomes in Developed Countries."

105   **In fact, as I mentioned:** Stanley Ip et al., "A Summary of the Agency for Healthcare Research and Quality's Evidence Report on Breastfeeding in Developed Countries," *Breastfeeding Medicine* 4, no. 1 (2009): S24.

105   **Drawing on other research:** Eidelman and Schanler, "Breastfeeding and the Use of Human Milk," e830.

105   **the AHRQ meta-analysis stated:** Ip et al., "A Summary of the Agency for Healthcare Research," S17.

105   **Turning next to the PROBIT study:** Eidelman and Schanler, "Breastfeeding and the Use of Human Milk," e830.

105   **It made no mention:** Interview with Schanler, August 6, 2014.

106   **It serves as the basis for:** Eidelman and Schanler, "Breastfeeding and the Use of Human Milk," e827.

106   **The report states clearly that:** Ibid.

107   **"Assess if breastfeeding . . . needed for the feeding":** "New York City Health Department Launches 'Latch On NYC' Initiative to Support Breastfeeding Mothers," New York City Department of Health and Mental Hygiene, May 9, 2010, www .nyc.gov/html/doh/html/pr2012/pr013-12.shtml.

107   **Latch On NYC also includes:** "NYSDOH Breastfeeding Quality Improvement in Hospitals (BQIH) Change Package," New York State Department of Health, September 2014.

107   **This way, the RN has to sign:** Mary Kay Linge, "Mayor Bloomberg Pushing NYC Hospitals to Hide Baby Formula So

More New Moms Will Breast-Feed," *New York Post*, July 29, 2012.

107   **A blogger on the popular . . . mothers for bottlefeeding"**: Esti commenting online at Caperton, "Latch On, NYC—OR ELSE," Feministe, August 31, 2012, www.feministe.us/blog/archives /2012/07/31/latch-on-nyc-or-else/.

109   **More than half the babies**: USDA Food and Nutrition Service, "About WIC: WIC at a Glance," US Department of Agriculture, February 2015, www.fns.usda.gov/wic/about-wic-wic-glance.

109   **In 2014, a family of two**: USDA Food and Nutrition Service, "WIC Income Eligibility Guidelines," US Department of Agriculture, February 2015, www.fns.usda.gov/wic/wic-income -eligibility-guidelines.

109   **But they have much more**: Some of these mothers are black (19 percent) or Hispanic (39 percent), many are white (35 percent), and all of them are poor. These percentages are drawn from Centers for Disease Control and Prevention, "Eligibility and Enrollment in the Special Supplemental Nutrition Program for Women, Infants, and Children (WIC)—27 States and New York City, 2007–2008," *Morbidity and Mortality Weekly Report* 63, no. 10 (March 2013): 189–193.

110   **Since 1998, WIC has been required**: USDA Food and Nutrition Service, "Legislative History of Breastfeeding Promotion Requirements in WIC," US Department of Agriculture, November 2013, www.fns.usda.gov/wic/about-wic-wic-glance, www.fns.usda.gov/wic/breastfeeding/bflegishistory.HTM.

111   **Among other things, it allowed**: Every Mother, Inc., "Using Loving Support to Grow and Glow in WIC: Breastfeeding Training for Local WIC Staff," in cooperation with USDA, 2007, http://everymother.org/training_programs.php.

111   **For me, the most outrageous feature**: https://s3.amazonaws .com/aws.upl/nwica.org/breastfeeding_infographic2013.pdf.

111   **The enhanced food package**: HHS, *The Surgeon General's Call to Action*, 20.

111   **Infants who are breastfed**: "The New WIC: Food and Focus Breastfeeding," Missouri Department of Health and Senior Services, June 2, 2009. This is from a two-page educational handout provided to new mothers at WIC clinics in Missouri. The educational material was adapted from a similar handout provided in Colorado. Health.mo.gov/living/families/.../LWPB FFFoodPkgEducation.doc.

111   **Fully breastfeeding mothers get:** Ibid.

111   **A mother who requests formula:** Ibid.

112   **Babies who are fully breastfed are:** Ibid.

112   **"We don't make . . . breastfeeding food package":** Interview
      with Cheryl Lauth, director of WIC for Catholic Charities of
      Western New York, October 29, 2014.

113   **Often it's the same course:** Caperton, "Latch On, NYC—OR
      ELSE."

114   **Joining one conversation . . . I had to supplement":** Nicole,
      "Am I the only one who feels this way (wic and breastfeeding)?"
      Yahoo! Answers, June 4, 2010, http://answers.yahoo.com
      /question/index?qid=20100604144306AA2kRTZ.

114   **Another mother chimed in . . . poison or something":** Ibid.

115   **"In my experience . . . paying for food":** Caperton, "Latch On,
      NYC—OR ELSE."

115   **Another mother recalled:** Interview with Kim Taylor, October
      2014, Odessa, Texas.

115   **It goes on and on:** (mint, August 23, 2011 http://wicwoes.com
      /2011/wic-moms-dont-breastfeed#comment-2234. Source
      material available in print from author; Caperton, "Latch On,
      NYC—OR ELSE."

115   **I got yelled at by wic:** Elizabeth P., "Why do people hate on
      mothers who receive WIC?" Yahoo! Answers, June 25, 2008,
      http://answers.yahoo.com/question/index?qid=200801242
      10954AAUagip.

115   **That data reveals that:** For 2007 data, see "Provisional
      Breastfeeding Rates by Socio-Demographic Factors, Among
      Children Born in 2007 (Percent +/–half 95% Confidence
      Interval)," National Immunization Survey, Centers for Disease
      Control and Prevention (CDC), Department of Health and
      Human Services (HHS), www.cdc.gov/breastfeeding/data/NIS
      _data/2007/socio-demographic_any.htm. For 2010 data, see
      "Rates of Any and Exclusive Breastfeeding by Socio-
      Demographics Among Children Born in 2010 (Percentage
      +/–half 95% Confidence Interval)," National Immunization
      Survey, CDC, HHS, www.cdc.gov/breastfeeding/data/nis_data
      /rates-any-exclusive-bf-socio-dem-2010.htm.

116   **When the results of that survey:** Rachel Rettner, "Breastfeeding
      Rate Has Increased but Few Mothers Are Nursing for
      Recommended Time," Huffington Post, March 15, 2013, http://

www.huffingtonpost.com/2013/02/07/breastfeeding-rate-has
-in_n_2639043.html.

116 **The CDC acknowledges that:** "More Mothers Are Breastfeeding:
African American Mothers Need More Support," Centers for
Disease Control and Prevention, Department of Health and
Human Services, www.cdc.gov/media/releases/2013/p0207
_breast_feeding.html.

116 **Readers are told only that:** US Department of Health and
Human Services (HHS), *An Easy Guide to Breastfeeding for
African American Women* (Washington, DC: HHS, Office on
Women's Health, 2006), 4.

116 **Finally, the guide warns:** Ibid., 25.

117 **A voice-over describes:** A description of the ad, and of the
controversy it sparked at the time, can be found here: Tatiana
Morales, "Battle over Breastfeeding Ads," *CBS,* December 13,
2003, www.cbsnews.com/2100–500165_162–590864.html.

117 **The ad sparked outrage:** Ibid.

117 **Critics argued that the ad:** Marc Kaufman and Christopher Lee,
"HHS Toned Down Breast-Feeding Ads," *Washington Post* Staff
Writers, August 31, 2007, http://www.washingtonpost.com
/wp-dyn/content/article/2007/08/30/AR2007083002198.html;
Suzanne Barston, "The Bull(shit) That Wouldn't Die: The 2003
DHHS Breastfeeding Ad Rears Its Ugly Head," Fearless Formula
Feeder, May 2, 2011, www.fearlessformulafeeder.com/2011/05
/the-bullshit-that-wouldnt-die-the-2003-dhhs-breastfeeding
-ad-rears-its-ugly-head/.

119 **The comparatively low breastfeeding:** Theola Labbe Dubose,
"Program Seeks to Increase Breast-Feeding Among Black
Women in District," *Washington Post,* January 2, 2012, 5;
Jennifer Ludden, "Teaching Black Women to Embrace Breast-
Feeding," *National Public Radio,* December 23, 2009; Barbara L.
Philipp and Sheina Jean-Marie, *African American Women and
Breastfeeding* (Washington, DC: Joint Center for Political and
Economic Studies Health Policy Institute, 2007).

119 **Those studies routinely show:** Philipp and Jean-Marie, *African
American Women and Breastfeeding,* 5.

119 **Efforts to explain this preference:** Centers for Disease Control
and Prevention, "Racial and Ethnic Differences in Breastfeeding
Initiation and Duration, by State—National Immunization
Survey, United States, 2004–2008," *Weekly Morbidity Report* 59,
no. 11 (March 26, 2010): 327–334.

119   **For one thing, although they have:** Laura E. Caulfield, "WIC-Based Interventions to Promote Breastfeeding Among African American Women in Baltimore: Effects on Breastfeeding Initiation and Continuation," *Journal of Human Lactation* 14, no. 1 (March 1998): 15–22, jhl.sagepub.com/content/14/1/15.short ?rss=1&ssource=mfc.

120   **Even New York City's Latch On:** Interview with Dr. Thomas Farley, August 5, 2014, New York City.

120   **According to Blum:** Linda M. Blum, *At the Breast: Ideologies of Breastfeeding and Motherhood in the Contemporary United States* (Boston: Beacon Press, 1999), 152.

120   **Breastfeeding, they feel:** Ibid., 163.

120   **In the interviews Blum conducted:** Ibid., 164–169. Many of Blum's findings are corroborated by a breastfeeding counselor working with African American women, who explained why the women she worked with refused to breastfeed. See the African American lactivist website called Blacktating: Sarah Hill, "Guest Post: Breastfeeding Counselor Chronicles: African-American Moms," Blacktating, July 20, 2010, www.blacktating.com/2010 /07/guest-post-breastfeeding-counselor.html.

121   **The American health-care industry:** Steven Brill, *America's Bitter Pill: Money, Politics, Back-Room Deals, and the Fight to Fix Our Broken Healthcare System* (New York: Random House, 2015).

121   **Meanwhile the cost of health care:** Center for Consumer Information and Insurance Oversight, "Affordable Care Act Requires Insurance Companies to Justify High Rate Hikes," Centers for Medicare and Medicaid Services, December 21, 2010, www.cms.gov/CCIIO/Resources/Fact-Sheets-and-FAQs /ratereview.html.

121   **A 2012 poll revealed:** "Health Care Statistics," Health Care Problems, March 3, 2015, www.healthcareproblems.org/health -care-statistics.htm.

121   **Even after the Affordable Care Act:** Brill, *America's Bitter Pill.*

121   **The CDC reports that:** Centers for Disease Control and Prevention, "Chronic Diseases and Health Promotion," National Center for Chronic Disease Prevention and Health Promotion, May 9, 2014, www.cdc.gov/nccdphp/overview.htm.

122   **The DHHS and the CDC:** Ibid.

122   **For many years, smoking:** Siddhartha Mukherjee, *The Emperor of All Maladies: A Biography of Cancer* (New York: Scribner, 2011).

122   **In January 2013 ScienceDaily:** Florida Atlantic University,
      "Obesity Approaching Cigarette Smoking as Leading Avoidable
      Cause of Premature Deaths Worldwide," ScienceDaily, January
      31, 2013, www.sciencedaily.com/releases/2013/01/130131083755
      .htm.
122   **"at the rate we're going:** R. Morgan Griffin, "Obesity Epidemic
      'Astronomical,'" WebMD, 2013, www.webmd.com/diet/features
      /obesity-epidemic-astronomical.

CHAPTER 5

129   **An instructional video:** "How to Use Hands Free Pump Bra,"
      YouTube Video, 1:43, posted by "handsfreepumpbra," January
      26, 2010, www.youtube.com/watch?v=TS83BjAnXT0.
131   **One study found that 85 percent:** Judith Labiner-Wolfe et al.,
      "Prevalence of Breast Milk Expression and Associated Factors,"
      Pediatrics 122, no. S2 (October 2008): S63.
131   **Medela, one of the leading manufacturers:** Michael Johnsen,
      "Breastfeeding Grows into Destination Category," *Drug Store
      News* 30, no. 6 (May 19, 2008): 52.
131   **Amanda Cole, the owner of:** Interview with Amanda Cole,
      August 6, 2014, New York City.
131   **Twenty-five percent of breastfeeding:** Labiner-Wolfe et al.,
      "Prevalence of Breast Milk Expression and Associated Factors,"
      S63–S68.
131   **Most women who pump:** Ibid.
131   **These percentages translate:** Joyce A. Martin et al., "Births:
      Final Data for 2012," *National Vital Statistics Report* 62, no. 9
      (December 2013): 1–68.
132   **Seventy-nine percent (3.1 million):** Centers for Disease Control
      and Prevention, "Breastfeeding Report Card—United States,
      2012," Department of Health and Human Services, August 2012,
      www.cdc.gov/breastfeeding/pdf/2012breastfeedingreportcard.pdf.
132   **One apparently small subset:** Kathleen M. Rasmussen and
      Sheila Geraghty, "The Quiet Revolution: Breastfeeding
      Transformed with the Use of Breast Pumps," *American Journal of
      Public Health* 101, no. 8 (August 2011): 1356–1359.
132   **The number of EPs is high:** Jen, Amy, and Christine, "Exclusive
      Pumping Rules" (blog), Blogspot, http://pumpingrules.blog
      spot.ca.

133   **In fact, a 2006 study showed:** Alan S. Ryan et al., "The Effect of Employment Status on Breastfeeding in the United States," *Women's Health Issues* 16, no. 5 (September 2006): 243–251.

133   **An earlier study:** Sara B. Fein and Brian Roe, "The Effect of Work Status on Initiation and Duration of Breast-Feeding," *American Journal of Public Health* 88, no. 7 (July 1998): 1043.

133   **"Full-time working mothers:** Ibid., 1044.

133   **A more recent study:** Chinelo Ogbuanu et al., "The Effect of Maternity Leave Length and Time of Return to Work on Breastfeeding," *Pediatrics* 127, no. 6 (June 2011): e1414–e1427.

134   **Instead, "approximately 14%:** US Department of Health and Human Services (HHS), *The Surgeon General's Call to Action to Support Breastfeeding* (Washington, DC: HHS, Office of the Surgeon General, 2011), 30.

134   **Fourteen percent of management:** Ibid.

135   **That number also differs by race:** US Department of Health and Human Services (HHS), Health Resources and Services Administration, Maternal and Child Health Bureau, *Women's Health USA 2011* (Rockville, MD: HHS, 2011), www.mchb.hrsa .gov/whusa11/hstat/hsrmh/pages/233ml.html.

136   **In fact, the Department of Health:** US Department of Health and Human Services (HHS), Health Resources and Services Administration, Maternal and Child Health Bureau, *The Business Case for Breastfeeding* (Rockville, MD: HHS, 2008), http://mchb.hrsa.gov/pregnancyandbeyond/breastfeeding/.

136   **You would be shocked at the places:** "Thread: VENTING pumping at work difficulties!" Many users post personal experiences on La Leche League International's online forum (June 2013), http://forums.llli.org/showthread.php?117302 -VENTING-pumping-at-work-diffiuculties!; "Working and Breastfeeding," La Leche League online forum, http://forums .llli.org/forumdisplay.php?39-Working-and-Breastfeeding.

137   **In a publication designed for:** HHS, *The Business Case for Breastfeeding*, 3.

137   **Many say that coworkers have:** Shawna Cohen, "The Secret World of Videotaping Women as They Pump Breast Milk," Mommyish, June 6, 2012, www.mommyish.com/2012/06/06 /the-secret-world-of-videotaping-women-as-they-pump -breast-milk-696/#ixzz3TRyyykb9.

137 **A couple of women:** "Cops: Man Hid Camera to Film Breast Pumping," The Smoking Gun, June 1, 2012, www.thesmoking gun.com/documents/bizarre/man-secretly-filmed-breast feeding-coworker-798435.

137 **To avoid some of these risks:** Katherine Lewis, "Mom-Tested Techniques to Increase Your Milk Supply," About.com, accessed March 4, 2015, http://workingmoms.about.com/od/todayswork ingmoms/a/pumpingtips.htm; "Pumping and Driving," online forum, Baby Center, March 2012, http://community.babycenter .com/post/a32102629/driving_and_pumping.

139 **As her milk supply dwindled:** Andrew R. MacIlvane, "The ACA and Nursing Mothers," Human Resource Executive Online, February 3, 2014, www.hreonline.com/HRE/view/story.jhtml ?id=534356662.

139 **In fact, the La Leche League:** "Working and Breastfeeding," La Leche League online forum, http://forums.llli.org/forumdisplay .php?39-Working-and-Breastfeeding.

139 **Many working mothers:** Colorado Breastfeeding Coalition, http://cobfc.org.

139 **Almost every woman I have:** See http://cobfc.org for videos of women who describe these experiences. For accounts of resentful coworkers, see Linda Szmulewitz, "Pumping at Work: One Mom's Frustrating Story," The Chicago New Moms Group, November 10, 2011, http://chicagonewmomsgroup.com /pumping-at-work.

140 **But jokes about pumping:** "Working and Breastfeeding," La Leche League online forum, http://forums.llli.org/forumdisplay .php?39-Working-and-Breastfeeding.

140 **As the Department of Health:** HHS, *The Business Case for Breastfeeding*, 5.

140 **Notwithstanding its stern pronouncement:** National Conference of State Legislatures, "Breastfeeding State Laws," Maternal and Child Health Bureau (Title V, Social Security Act), Health Resources and Services Administration, US Department of Health and Human Services, March 31, 2015, www.ncsl.org /issues-research/health/breastfeeding-state-laws.aspx.

141 **But the department decided:** Wage and Hour Division, US Department of Labor, "Reasonable Break Time for Nursing Mothers," *WHD Notices* 75, no. 244, December 21, 2010, http://

webapps.dol.gov/FederalRegister/HtmlDisplay.aspx?DocId
=24540&Month=12&Year=2010.

141　**But it cannot levy any fine:** Allison Yarrow, "Pumped Up:
Breastfeeding Mothers Fight for Rights at Work," *NBC News,*
January 10, 2014, http://usnews.nbcnews.com/_news/2014/01
/10/22257760-pumped-up-breastfeeding-mothers-fight-for
-rights-at-work%23th3916076-c81602662.

141　**A small number of women:** Galen Sherwin, "Nationwide
Nursing Mom Told at Office to 'Just Go Home,'" American Civil
Liberties Union of Iowa, Women's Rights Project, April 29, 2014,
www.aclu-ia.org/2014/04/21/nationwide-nursing-mom-told-to
-just-go-home/.

142　**Then she handed Ames:** "Brief of the Equal Employment
Opportunity Commission as Amicus Curiae in Support of
Plaintiff Angela Ames," *Angela Ames v. Nationwide Insurance Co.,*
Nationwide Advantage Mortgage Co., and Karla Neel, No.
12–3780 (8th Cir. 2003), www.eeoc.gov/eeoc/litigation/briefs
/ames.html.

142　**Some months later, Ames:** NCTBA.org, "Breastfeeding Mother
Quits Job, Files Civil Rights Complaint," Triangle Breastfeeding
Alliance, October 6, 2010, www.nctba.org/breastfeeding/breast
feeding-mother-quits-job-files-civil-rights-complaint.

142　**The EEOC thought that:** Jacob Gershman, "Appeals Court Rules
Against Breastfeeding Employee Who Claimed Discrimination,"
Law Blog, *Wall Street Journal,* May 17, 2014, http://blogs.wsj
.com/law/2014/03/17/appeals-court-rules-against-breastfeeding
-employee-who-claimed-discrimination/.

142　**The lawsuit was dismissed:** Nicole Flatow, "Woman Whose Boss
Told Her 'It's Best You Go Home with Your Babies' Won't Get
Discrimination Trial," ThinkProgress, March 19, 2014, http://
thinkprogress.org/justice/2014/03/19/3416008/employee
-who-was-told-its-best-you-go-home-with-your-babies-wont
-get-discrimination-trial/.

142　**The somewhat incredible reasoning:** Ibid.

143　**In June 2014:** Abigail Rubenstein, "Breastfeeding Ruling Botched
Sex-Stereotyping, 8th Circ. Told," Law360, April 30, 2014, www
.law360.com/articles/533233/breastfeeding-ruling-botched-sex
-stereotyping-8th-circ-told.; Vin Gurrieri, "8th Circ. Won't
Rehear Worker's Breastfeeding Bias Case," Law360, June 26,
2014, www.law360.com/articles/552165/8th-circ-won-t

-rehear-worker-s-breastfeeding-bias-case?article_related
_content=1.

143   **In 2011, the IRS amended:** Tom Murse, "Are Breast Pumps
Tax Deductible?" About.com, accessed March 3, 2015, http://
usgovinfo.about.com/od/healthcare/a/Breast-Pumps-Tax
-Deductible.htm.

143   **To be clear, that does not mean:** Kristin Wartman, "Tea Partiers
Milk Anger over Breastfeeding," Civil Eats, February 22, 2011,
http://civileats.com/2011/02/22/tea-partiers-milk-anger-over
-breastfeeding/.

144   **When I asked him about:** E-mail exchange with Steven Brill,
February 3, 2015.

144   **What free breast pumps mean:** "What Am I Eligible For?"
Insurance Orders, Yummy Mummy: All Things Breastfeeding,
http://yummymummystore.com/insurance/eligibility.

145   **Whereas the most popular pumps:** Deborah Kotz, "Demand
for Breast Pumps Surge with New Coverage Under Health Law,"
Boston Globe Online, January 15, 2013, www.boston.com/daily
dose/2013/01/15/demand-for-breast-pumps-surge-with-new
-coverage-under-health-law/vpKgXHHkQNiu5sgs7Ir9BK/story
.html.

145   **In 2010, Medela claimed:** UHY International, "Medela AG
Medical Technology," UHY Capability Statement (2011), www
.uhy.com/wp-content/uploads/UHY-Medela-AG-Case-Study
-Port.pdf.

146   **By 2015, the worldwide market:** Jessica Grose, "Working Moms
Need More Than Subsidized Breast Pumps," Bloomberg Business
Online, February 7, 2013, www.bloomberg.com/bw/articles
/2013-02-07/working-moms-need-more-than-subsidized-breast
-pumps.

CHAPTER 6

149   **By invoking the authority:** Marc Kaufman and Christopher
Lee, "HHS Toned Down Breast-Feeding Ads," *Washington Post*
Staff Writers, August 31, 2007, http://www.washingtonpost.com
/wp-dyn/content/article/2007/08/30/AR2007083002198.html.

149   **"We were thinking of breast milk:** Interview with Dr. Thomas
Farley, August 5, 2014, New York City.

151   **In case you're wondering:** University of Western Australia,
School of Chemistry and Biochemistry, Human Lactation

Research Group, www.chembiochem.uwa.edu.au/research
/human-lactation.

151 **In 1993, the ILCA convened:** Linda J. Smith, *The Lactation
Consultant in Private Practice: The ABC's of Getting Started*
(Sudbury, MA: Jones and Bartlett, 2003).

152 **In fact, many women who were already:** Interview with Edith
White Fletcher, September 19, 2014.

155 **He presented his work:** Medela's 8th Breastfeeding and
Lactation Symposium, Copenhagen, April 13, 2013, www
.medela.com/IW/en/breastfeeding/about-medela/media
/global-press-releases/medela-8th-bf-symposium.html.

156 **It came from a breast-pump manufacturer:** Telephone
interview with Dr. Richard Schanler, August 6, 2014.

156 **I asked Schanler if he:** Ibid.

156 **His background in breastfeeding:** Telephone interview with Dr.
Richard Schanler, June 1, 2015.

157 **From Dr. Schanler's perspective:** Ibid.

157 **According to Chief Executive Officer:** Andrew Pollack, "Breast
Milk Becomes a Commodity, with Mothers Caught Up in
Debate," *New York Times*, March 20, 2015.

158 **At one dollar per ounce:** "Find a Milk Bank," Prolacta
Bioscience, accessed March 4, 2015, www.prolacta.com/find
-a-milk-bank.

158 **Many breastfeeding advocates:** Amy, "Swindled: The Ugly Side
of Milk Donations," JustWestofCrunchy (blog), June 23, 2011,
http://amywest.co/2011/06/23/swindled-the-ugly-side-of-milk
-donation-prolacta.

158 **In 2013 and 2014, two of the three:** Amy B. Hair et al.,
"Randomized Trial of Human Milk Cream as a Supplement to
Standard Fortification of an Exclusive Human Milk–Based Diet
in Infants 750–1250 g Birth Weight," *Journal of Pediatrics* 165,
no. 5 (November 2014): 915–920, doi:10.1016/j.jpeds.2014
.07.005; E. A. Cristofalo et al., "Randomized Trial of Exclusive
Human Milk Versus Preterm Formula Diets in Extremely
Premature Infants," *Journal of Pediatrics* 163, no. 6 (December
2013): 1592–1595, doi:10.1016/j.jpeds.2013.07.011; S. A. Abrams
et al., "Greater Mortality and Morbidity in Extremely Preterm
Infants Fed a Diet Containing Cow Milk Protein Products,"
Breastfeeding Medicine 9, no. 6 (July/August 2014): 281–2815,
doi: 10.1089/bfm.2014.0024; see also www.prolacta.com

/publications-1 for a list of Prolacta publications as of April 2015.

158 **Ironically, one of them, Ernie Strapazon:** "Board of Directors," Prolacta Bioscience, March 2015, www.prolacta.com/board-of -directors.

158 **Those papers were all published:** Sandra Sullivan et al., "An Exclusively Human Milk–Based Diet Is Associated with a Lower Rate of Necrotizing Enterocolitis Than a Diet of Human Milk and Bovine Milk–Based Products," *Journal of Pediatrics* 56, no. 4 (April 2010): 562–567.

161 **In 2011, the *New York Times*:** Nicholas Bakalar, "Breast Milk Donated or Sold Online Is Often Tainted, Study Says," *New York Times,* Health Section, October 21, 2013.

161 **But there are only twenty-two:** "Locations," Human Milk Banking Association of North America, accessed March 2015, www.hmbana.org/locations.

162 **Three Internet samples:** Sarah A. Keim et al., "Microbial Contamination of Human Milk Purchased via the Internet," *Pediatrics* 132, no. 5 (August 2013):e1227–35, http://pediatrics .aappublications.org/content/early/2013/10/16/peds.2013-1687 .full.pdf.

162 **Follow-up research, published:** Nicholas Bakalar, "Online Breast Milk May Contain Cow's Milk," *New York Times*, April 6, 2015.

163 **And obviously milk bought:** Bakalar, "Breast Milk Donated or Sold Online Is Often Tainted."

164 **But just in case, they:** "The Four Pillars of Safe Breast Milk Sharing," Eats on Feets, accessed March 5, 2015, www.eats onfeets.org#fourPillars.

164 **This group uses "social media:** Quote from home page, Human Milk 4 Human Babies, accessed March 5, 2015, http://hm4hb .net.

164 **The women posting anonymously:** HM4HB Connecticut Facebook webpage: www.facebook.com/hm4hbConnecticut.

165 **They want "milk sharing and wet-nursing:** Ibid.

165 **Their website states that:** Ibid.

166 **"It's hard for me . . . psychosocial benefit there":** Interview with Dr. Thomas Farley, August 5, 2014, New York City.

167 **That report found:** Stanley Ip et al., "A Summary of the Agency for Healthcare Research and Quality's Evidence Report on

Breastfeeding in Developed Countries," *Breastfeeding Medicine* 4, no. 1 (2009): S17.

168   **He also likes to cite:** Interview with Dr. Michael S. Kramer, December 12, 2013, Montreal, Canada.

168   **So we know enough about:** Ibid.

169   **Apparently some research:** Kathleen M. Rasmussen and Sheela Geraghty, "The Quiet Revolution: Breastfeeding Transformed with the Use of Breast Pumps," *American Journal of Public Health* 101, no. 8 (August 2011): 1356–1359.

169   **"At a minimum," says the:** Ibid.

CHAPTER 7

175   **As early as 1983, researchers:** "History of AIDS Up to 1986," AVERT, December 12, 2014, www.avert.org/history-aids-1986 .htm.

175   **In 1985, two thousand activists:** Ibid.

175   **Even in the United States:** Philip Boffey, "AIDS in the Future: Experts Say Deaths Will Climb Sharply," *New York Times,* January 14, 1986.

176   **In the countries of East and Southern Africa:** By 1989, 30 percent of pregnant women in the Ugandan capital of Kampala were infected with HIV. In 2010, over 30 percent of women who attended public health sector clinics in South Africa were HIV positive. See Peter Barron et al., "Eliminating Mother-to-Child Transmission in South Africa," *Bulletin of the World Health Organization* 91, no. 1 (2013): 70–74.

176   **WHO and UNICEF estimated that:** WHO/UNAIDS, *A Review of HIV Transmission Through Breastfeeding: UNICEF, UNAIDS, WHO HIV and Infant Feeding* (WHO/UNAIDS, December 1998), 6, www.unaids.org/sites/default/files/media_asset/jc 180-hiv-infantfeeding-3_en_3.pdf.

177   **Between 1994 and 1997, the number:** IRIN, "Namibia: HIV/ AIDS Eats into Progress on Infant Mortality," IRIN News, July 28, 1999, www.irinnews.org/report/8300/namibia-hiv-aids-eats -into-progress-on-infant-mortality.

177   **In 2000, experts projected:** UNAIDS/UNICEF, "HIV/AIDS," United Nations Special Session on Children, May 2002, www .unicef.org/specialsession/about/sgreport-pdf/21_HIV-AIDS _D7341Insert_English.pdf.

177   **In the twenty-five years since 1990:** In 1997, the specific figure
was 600,000, according to Michael Specter, "Weighing Health
Risks," *New York Times,* August 19, 1998. In 2008, it was 430,000,
according to the World Health Organization. Because of the
increasing use of antiretrovirals, that number was over half a
million in the 1990s and under half a million in the 2000s. In
2011, it was 330,000—a significant achievement.

177   **Nine out of ten children infected:** "Children, HIV and AIDS,"
AVERT, July 30, 2014, www.avert.org/children-and-hiv-aids.htm.

177   **The fetus may contract HIV in utero:** Michael Carter, "Mother-
to-Baby Transmission," NAM/Aidsmap, August 8, 2011, www
.aidsmap.com/Mother-to-baby-transmission/page/1044918.

177   **The crucial 1985 article that:** John B. Ziegler et al., "Postnatal
Transmission of AIDS-Associated Retrovirus from Mother to
Infant," *The Lancet* 325, no. 8434 (April 1985): 896–898; John B.
Ziegler et al., "Breastfeeding During Primary Maternal
Immunodeficiency Virus Infection and Risk of Transmission
from Mother to Infant," *Journal of Infectious Disease* 167, no. 2
(1993): 441–444; Philippe Van de Perre et al., "Postnatal
Transmission of Human Immunodeficiency Virus Type 1 from
Mother to Infant: A Prospective Cohort Study in Kigali,
Rwanda," *New England Journal of Medicine* 325, no. 9 (August
1991): 593–598; E. Richard Stiehm and Peter Vink,
"Transmission of Human Immunodeficiency Virus Infection by
Breastfeeding," *Journal of Pediatrics* 118, no. 3 (March 1991):
410–412; S. K. Hira et al., "Apparent Vertical Transmission of
Human Immunodeficiency Virus Type 1 by Breast-Feeding in
Zambia," *Journal of Pediatrics* 117, no. 3 (September 1990):
421–424; Robert Colebunders et al., "Breastfeeding and
Transmission of HIV," *The Lancet* 332, no. 8626–8627
(December 1988): 1487; Philippe Lepage et al., "Postnatal
Transmission of HIV from Mother to Child," *The Lancet* 330, no.
8555 (August 1987): 400; R. W. Nduati et al., "Postnatal
Transmission of HIV-1 Through Pooled Breast Milk," *The Lancet*
344, no. 8934 (November 19, 1994): 1432.

177   **Not only had medical testing shown:** WHO/UNAIDS, *A
Review of HIV Transmission Through Breastfeeding,* 8.

177   **Research also showed that:** Ibid., 14.

178   **This new test made it:** Martha F. Rogers et al., "Use of the
Polymerase Chain Reaction for Early Detection of the Proviral
Sequences of Human Immunodeficiency Virus in Infants Born

to Seropositive Mothers," *New England Journal of Medicine* 320, no. 25 (June 22, 1989): 1649–1654; see also "HIV and Breastfeeding," AVERT, December 12, 2014, www.avert.org w/hiv-and-breastfeeding.htm.

178   **In 1992, *The Lancet* published:** D. T. Dunn et al., "Risk of Human Immunodeficiency Virus Type 1 Transmission Through Breastfeeding," *The Lancet* 340, no. 8819 (September 5, 1992): 585–588; see also "HIV and Breastfeeding."

178   **Following the 1985 discovery that:** Centers for Disease Control and Prevention, "Recommendation for Assisting in the Prevention of Perinatal Transmission of Human T Lymphotropic Virus Type III/Lymphadenopathy-Associated Virus and Acquired Immunodeficiency Syndrome," *Morbidity and Mortality Weekly Report* 34, no. 721 (1985); Lawrence M. Gartner et al., "Breastfeeding and the Use of Human Milk," American Academy of Pediatrics Section on Breastfeeding, *Pediatrics* 115, no. 2 (February 2005): 496–506.

179   **Many of them refused to believe:** Interview with Edith White Fletcher, September 19, 2014, via Skype.

180   **It didn't develop an official policy:** G. K. Howell et al., "Breastfeeding Promotion in WIC and HIV Infection: Policy Development Process," *Journal of the American Dietetic Association* 99, no. 9 (September 1999).

180   **In a phone conversation, the director:** Telephone interview with Cheryl Lauth, October 29, 2014.

182   **And so in 1987 WHO issued:** WHO, "Summary Statement on Breast-feeding/Breast Milk and Human Immunodeficiency Virus (HIV)," July 1, 1987; see also "HIV and Breastfeeding."

182   **In its 1987 Global AIDS Plan:** Ibid.

182   **In its 1989 report *State of the World's Children*:** James P. Grant, *State of the World's Children 1989* (New York: UNICEF, 1989).

183   **As Dr. Francis Miro, the beleaguered chief:** Michael Specter, "Breast-Feeding and H.I.V.: Weighing Health Risks and Treatment Costs," *New York Times*, August 19, 1998.

184   **Those studies uniformly concluded:** James G. Kahn et al., "Feeding Strategies for Children of HIV-Infected Mothers: Modeling the Trade-Off Between HIV Infection and Non-HIV Mortality," in Harris Kaplan and Ron Brookmeyer, eds., *Quantitative Evaluation of HIV Prevention Programs* (New Haven, CT: Yale University Press, 2002), 203.

184   **The weight of the evidence:** Ibid.

184 **As White deomonstrated starkly in her book:** Edith White, *Breastfeeding and HIV/AIDS: The Research, the Politics, the Women's Responses* (Jefferson, NC: McFarland, 1999).

184 **In 1993, UNICEF's *State of the World's Children*:** WHO/UNAIDS, *A Review of HIV Transmission Through Breastfeeding*, 6.

184 **UNICEF also published a report:** White, *Breastfeeding and HIV/AIDS*, 134.

185 **That book discussed the transmission:** Randa Saadeh et al., eds., *Breast-Feeding: The Technical Basis for Action* (Geneva, Switzerland: WHO, 1993).

185 **One 1995 study reported that:** Mansour Al-Nozha et al., "Horizontal Versus Vertical Transmission of Human Immunodeficiency Virus Type 1 (HIV-1): Experience from Southwestern Saudi Arabia," *Tropical and Geographical Medicine* 47, no. 6 (1995): 293–295.

185 **Similar studies reported rates:** Rachana Kumar et al., "A Prospective Study of Mother-to-Infant HIV Transmission in Tribal Women from India," *Journal of Acquired Immune Deficiency Syndromes & Human Retrovirology* 9, no. 3 (1995): 238–342; E. T. Taha et al., "The Effect of Human Immunodeficiency Virus Infection on Birthweight, and Infant and Child Mortality in Urban Malawi," *International Journal of Epidemiology* 24, no. 5 (1995): 1022–1029.

185 **The report also lamented the fact:** Carol Bellamy, *The State of the World's Children 1996* (New York: UNICEF/Oxford University Press, 1996).

185 **Although AIDS was the leading cause:** White, *Breastfeeding and HIV/AIDS*, 136.

185 **At the time, many scientists:** Barry Meier, "In War Against AIDS, Battle over Baby Formula Reignites," *New York Times*, June 8, 1997.

185 **In a 1998 interview with a:** White, *Breastfeeding and HIV/AIDS*, 132.

186 **That denial, she explained:** Ibid.

186 **Labbok has often publicly expressed:** Lawrence K. Altman, "AIDS Brings a Shift on Breastfeeding," *New York Times*, July 26, 1998; Anne McNulty, "Working for Healthy Mothers and Healthy Babies: Miriam Labbok, MD, MPH," UNC Institute for Global Health & Infectious Diseases, September 1, 2010, http://globalhealth.unc.edu/2010/09/working-for-healthy-mothers-and-healthy-babies-miriam-labbok-md-mph.

186 **A Zimbabwean delegate:** Interview with Fletcher, September 18, 2014.

186 **In a spectacular understatement:** Zarina Geloo, "HIV and Breastfeeding: Re-Igniting an Old Controversy," *Women's International Net Magazine*, 1998, in White, *Breastfeeding and HIV/AIDS*, 137.

186 **"Are we to accept that our children's:** Timothy Stamps, "Address to the World Health Assembly" (Geneva, Switzerland: WHO, May 1997), in White, *Breastfeeding and HIV/AIDS*, 130.

186 **"In the affluent industrialized countries:** Zorodzai Machekanyanga, "Zimbabwe: Is Breast Milk Still Best?," Harare, Zimbabwe: *Africa Information Afrique*, September 8, 1997, in White, *Breastfeeding and HIV/AIDS*, 137.

187 **In its major 1998 report on HIV transmission:** WHO/UNAIDS, *A Review of HIV Transmission Through Breastfeeding*.

187 **International health organizations finally acknowledged:** WHO/UNAIDS, *A Review of HIV Transmission Through Breastfeeding*.

187 **Nevertheless, according to a WHO report:** WHO/UNAIDS, *A Review of HIV Transmission Through Breastfeeding: A Review of Available Evidence, 2007 Update* (Geneva, Switzerland: WHO Press, 2008). See also http://wol.jw.org/en/wol/d/r1/lp-e/102000 007. UNICEF claimed that 500–700 children were infected every day through breastfeeding, which would put the annual figure at somewhere between 172,500 and 255,500.

188 **The statement also claimed:** Celia Farber, "HIV and Breastfeeding: The Fear. The Misconceptions. The Facts," *Mothering*, September/October 1998.

188 **A few months later, the February/March:** Maryanne Stone-Jimenez, "Mother-Child Transmission of HIV," *Leaven* 35, no.1 (February/March 1999): 3–5, www.lalecheleague.org/llleaderweb /lv/lvfebmar99p3.html.

188 **They concluded that "fear of HIV:** Maryanne Stone-Jimenez, "Mother-Child Transmission of HIV," *Leaven* 35, no. 1 (February/ March 1999): 3–5, www.lalecheleague.org/llleaderweb/lv/lvfeb mar99p3.html.

189 **David Crowe is a Canadian journalist:** As of March 2015 according to the Rethinking AIDS website, www.rethinkingaids .com/Content/TheBoard/tabid/60/Default.aspx.

189   **He is closely allied with Duesberg:** As listed on Rethinking AIDS 2011 tax return, available online: www.rethinkingaids.com /RA_Tax_Returns/RA_Tax_Return_2011.pdf.

190   **Crowe also provides medical advice:** M. Aziz, "Correspondence Between HIV+ Patient and David Crowe," Immunity Resource Foundation, May 29, 2014, www.immunity .org.uk/correspondence-hiv-patient-david-crowe/.

190   **A visit to the Reappraising AIDS website:** http://aras.ab.ca. Source material available in print from author. (This web-page is a constantly updated list of news items and commentary Crowe finds interesting. The claim that Ebola is a mythical virus is no longer on the page, but when I e-mailed Crowe about it he explained at considerable length why he believes Ebola is a mythical virus. E-mail exchange with David Crowe, April 15, 2015.

190   **He also had some more tangential:** E-mail exchange with David Crowe, April 15, 2015.

190   **He also alleged that the PCR test:** David Crowe, "Infectious HIV in Breastmilk: Fact or Fantasy?" La Leche League International Conference Session 205: Perspectives on HIV, AIDS and Breastfeeding Research, July 9, 2001, www.another look.org/presentations/LLLI-200107-factorfantasy.pdf.

190   **They could "accept current dogmas:** Ibid.

191   **a prominent antivaccine doctor:** Patricia Callahan and Trine Tsouderos, "Autism Doctor: Troubling Record Trailing Doctor Treating Autism," *Chicago Tribune,* May 22, 2009.

192   **One such presentation states:** Miles Cloyd, "Detecting Infectious HIV in Human Milk," Department of Immunology and Microbiology, University of Texas, July 2003, www.another look.org/presentations/LLLI-200307-detecting.pdf.

192   **Another proposes that many children:** George Kent, "HIV/ AIDS, Infant Feeding and Human Rights," University of Hawaii, July 2005, www.anotherlook.org/presentations/LLLI-200507 -infantfeedingandhumanrights.pdf.

192   **That same paper concludes:** Kent, "HIV/AIDS, Infant Feeding and Human Rights."

192   **Now in her capacity as a UNICEF:** Miriam Labbok, "Update on HIV and Breastfeeding in the Most Vulnerable Populations: Myths and Controversies," UNICEF, www.anotherlook.org /presentations/LLLI-200507-hivmyths.pdf.

193   *Mothering* **magazine also honored:** David Crowe, "AIDS and Breastfeeding," *Mothering,* April 2, 2012, www.mothering.com /articles/aids-and-breastfeeding.

193   **In fact, when I contacted La Leche League International:** E-mail exchange with Diana West, LLLI media contact and spokesperson, April 2015.

194   **Finally, West disclosed that:** E-mail exchange with Diana West, LLLI media contact and spokesperson, April 2015.

194   **The CDC officially uses "number of La Leche League Leaders...":** http://www.cdc.gov/breastfeeding/pdf/2014 breastfeedingreportcard.pdf.

195   **This rift routinely devolves:** Personal correspondence with Nicoli Nattrass, who has attended many such conferences in the course of conducting her research.

195   **Even when they are personally invited:** Penny van Esterik, a prominent figure in the world of breastfeeding research and advocacy and a well-respected professor at York University, had this experience when she convened a conference on breastfeeding and HIV at York. Organizers invited breastfeeding activists and AIDS researchers, but the latter refused the invitation. See, e.g., Penny van Esterik, "Breastfeeding and HIV/AIDS: Critical Gaps and Dangerous Intersections," in *Giving Breast Milk,* R. Shaw and A. Bartlett, eds. (Toronto: Demeter Press, 2010), 151–162.

195   **In 2010, it issued new guidelines:** WHO/UNAIDS, *Guidelines on HIV and Infant Feeding, 2010: Principles and Recommendations for Infant Feeding in the Context of HIV and a Summary of Evidence* (Geneva, Switzerland: WHO Press, 2010), http://whqlibdoc.who.int/publications/2010/9789241599535 _eng.pdf?ua=1.

196   **Even when ARVs are not available:** Ibid. 4.

196   **The contemporary WHO policy:** H. M. Coovadia et al., "Mother-to-Child Transmission of HIV-1 Infection During Exclusive Breastfeeding in the First 6 Months of Life: An Intervention Cohort Study," *The Lancet* 369, no. 9567 (March 31, 2007): 1107–1116; Coutsoudis et al. "Exclusive Breastfeeding and HIV," *AIDS* 16, Issue no. 3 (2002):498–499; "Method of Feeding and Transmission of HIV-1 from Mothers to Children by 15 Months of Age: Prospective Cohort Study from Durban South Africa," *AIDS* 15 (2001):379–387.

197   **Still, the best research on HIV:** Coovadia et al., "Mother-to-Child Transmission of HIV-1 Infection.

197   **In Mozambique, a very poor country:** "Young Child Survivial Development," www.unicef.org/mozambique/child_survival _2933.html.

197   **exclusive breastfeeding is not a cultural or traditional norm anywhere:** "Unfortunately, encouraging mothers to practice exclusive breastfeeding is far from easy. In most societies it is normal for a baby to be given water and other foods, as well as breast milk." See http://www.avert.org/hiv-and-breastfeeding .htm. Also in Coovadia et al., "Mother-to-Child Transmission of HIV-1 Infection."

198   **Pamela Morrison, an activist:** Pamela Morrison, "New HIV and Breastfeeding Resource from the World Alliance for Breastfeeding Action (WABA)," Lactation Matters, January 8, 2013, lactationmatters.org/2013/01/08/wabahivresource; Pamela Morrison et al., "Informed Choice in Infant Feeding Decisions Can Be Supported for Hiv-Infected Women Even in Industrialized Countries," AIDS 25, no. 15 (2011): 1807–1811.

198   **She uses that figure to support:** Morrison, "New HIV and Breastfeeding Resource from the World Alliance for Breastfeeding Action."

198   **In fact, researchers estimate:** Different studies have had different outcomes. See Grace John-Stewart, "Prevention of HIV Transmission During Breastfeeding in Resource-Limited Settings," UpToDate, September 28, 2012, www.uptodate.com /contents/prevention-of-hiv-transmission-during-breastfeeding -in-resource-limited-settings. UpToDate is an online resource for medical practitioners that provides a current review of all relevant medical literature on a particular topic.

198   **The most often cited study found that 2.2 percent:** As I mentioned above, studies have shown different results, and the variation appears to depend primarily on the viral load and CD4 count of the mother. If viral load is high and CD4 count is low, the risk of transmission, even with antiretrovirals, is higher. A summary of the relevant literature, including different findings for rates of transmission, has been written by Morrison, available at www.aidstar-one.com/sites/default/files/Table_of _Breastfeeding_Studies.pdf.

198   **Morrison confirmed to me that:** E-mail communication with Pamela Morrison, April 16, 2015.

198   **As Morrison explained to me:** Ibid.
198   **Most doctors and public health organizations:** E-mail exchange between Pamela Morrison and Dr. Michael Silverman, sent to me by Morrison, April, 16 and 19, 2015.
198   **Studies have shown that:** Arlene D. Bardeguez et al., "Adherence to Anti-retrovirals Among US Women During and After Pregnancy," *Journal of Acquired Immune Deficiency Syndromes* 48, no. 4 (August 1, 2008): 408–417.
199   **If the 2.2 percent figure:** Morrison, "New HIV and Breastfeeding Resource from the World Alliance for Breastfeeding Action."
199   **Mothers can also transmit potentially:** EarthTalk, "Does Mother's Milk Transfer Environmental Toxins to Breast-Feeding Babies?" *Scientific American,* January 26, 2010, www.scientific american.com/article.cfm?id=earth-talks-breast-feeding.
199   **Babies whose mothers have nutritional:** Eleni Roumeliotou, "How Maternal Diet and Lifestyle Affects the Nutritional Value of Breast Milk," GreenMedInfo, April 8, 2013, www.greenmed info.com/blog/how-maternal-diet-and-lifestyle-affects -nutritional-value-breast-milk; see also Lindsay H. Allen, "B Vitamins in Breast Milk: Relative Importance of Maternal Status and Intake, and Effects on Infant Status and Function," *Advances in Nutrition* 3, no. 3 (May 2012): 362–369.
199   **All breastfed babies are at risk:** Jonathon L. Maguire et al., "Association Between Total Duration of Breastfeeding and Iron Deficiency," *Pediatrics* 131, no. 5 (May 2013): e1530–e1537.

CONCLUSION

202   **Probably the best way to show:** "Norway: The WHO Code and Breastfeeding: An International Comparative Overview," Department of Health, Australian Government, May 3, 2012, www.health.gov.au/internet/publications/publishing.nsf/Content /int-comp-whocode-bf-init~int-comp-whocode-bf-init-ico~int -comp-whocode-bf-init-ico-norway.
202   **US versus Norway table:** 1. US numbers come from the CDC's National Immunization Survey: www.cdc.gov/breastfeeding /data/NIS_data/index.htm; 2. Norwegian numbers come from the US Department of Health and Human Services: www.health. gov.au/internet/publications/publishing.nsf/Content/int-comp

-whocode-bf-init~int-comp-whocode-bf-init-ico~int-comp
-whocode-bf-init-ico-norway.

203   **In the US, the most commonly cited:** Ruowei Li et al., "Why
      Mothers Stop Breastfeeding: Mothers' Self-Reported Reasons for
      Stopping During the First Year," *Pediatrics* 122, Suppl. 2
      (October 1, 2008): S69–S76.

203   **One study found that one in:** Alison Stuebe, "How Often Does
      Breastfeeding Come Undone?" Breastfeeding Medicine, http://
      bfmed.wordpress.com/2014/03/27/how-often-does-breast
      feeding-come-undone/#more-1181.

204   **Doctors estimate that up to 15 percent:** www.medscape.com
      /viewarticle/565620_4.

204   **As one breastfeeding advocate:** Stuebe, "How Often Does
      Breastfeeding Come Undone?"

204   **"A health care professional . . . various medical causes":**
      Marianne R. Neifert, "Prevention of Breastfeeding Tragedies,"
      Pediatric Clinics of North America 48, no. 2 (April 2001):
      273–297.

205   **The thread was started by:** https://m.facebook.com/notes
      /bottle-babies/the-insignificant-truth-about-women-who-cant
      -breastfeed/174242565987038/.

205   **She, too, finally learned:** Ibid.

211   **consider that the CDC website:** "Excessive Drinking Costs U.S.
      $223.5 Billion," Centers for Disease Control and Prevention,
      April 17, 2014, www.cdc.gov/features/alcoholconsumption
      /index.html.

212   **This may be because excessive:** Ibid.

Index

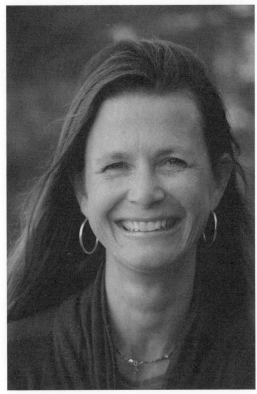

Courtney Jung is a professor in the Department of Political Science at the University of Toronto. She lives in Toronto, Ontario.